Autophagy

Discover How Fasting Heals Your Body, Fills It With Energy, And Clears Your Mind

By Peter Hardwood

© Copyright 2019 - All rights reserved.

The content contained within this book may not be reproduced, duplicated or transmitted without direct written permission from the author or the publisher.

Under no circumstances will any blame or legal responsibility be held against the publisher, or author, for any damages, reparation, or monetary loss due to the information contained within this book. Either directly or indirectly.

Legal Notice:

This book is copyright protected. This book is only for personal use. You cannot amend, distribute, sell, use, quote or paraphrase any part, or the content within this book, without the consent of the author or publisher.

Disclaimer Notice:

Please note the information contained within this document is for educational and entertainment purposes only. All effort has been executed to present accurate, up to date, and reliable, complete information. No warranties of any kind are declared or implied. Readers acknowledge that the author is not engaging in the rendering of legal, financial, medical or professional advice. The content within this book has been derived from various sources. Please consult a licensed professional before attempting any techniques outlined in this book.

By reading this document, the reader agrees that under no circumstances is the author responsible for any losses, direct or indirect, which are incurred as a result of the use of information contained within this document, including, but not limited to, — errors, omissions, or inaccuracies.

Table of Contents

Introduction 7

Part One - Autophagy 11

   History of Autophagy............................. 11

   What is Autophagy? 19

   What is mTOR, How It Affects the Autophagy and How to Balance It? 30

   Why is Autophagy Important and What Are Its Benefits? 38

Part Two – Inducing Autophagy........53

   Ketosis... 53

   Fasting.. 80
      History of Fasting 82
      How to Practice Intermittent Fasting 85

Part Three – Autophagy Without Fasting...108

   HIIT.. 108

   Protein Fast 115

Part Four – What You Will Need To Eat In Order To Induce Autophagy 123

   Types of Food Which Can Induce Autophagy 139

    Supplements Which Can Help You With Autophagy 144

Part Five – Changing Your Lifestyle . 151

    How To Make Fasting A Way of Life? ... 151

    Autophagy Without Fasting 165

Conclusion 175

References 178

Introduction

Have you ever wondered why humans today are affected by so many diseases? Have you wondered about the causes of these diseases? Today, the majority of diseases are caused by the food we eat, and this is mostly because of the high-carb intake we are exposed to.

Centuries ago, humans were not getting sick because of the food they were consuming; they were getting sick due to various other causes, but the low quality of food was not amongst those causes. If the medicine was not evolved back then, at least they had proper food, rich in nutritional value. Nowadays, we're experiencing the exact opposite of that situation. The medicine is more evolved than ever, but the food we are consuming has very low quality and little to nothing nutritional value. What happened in the meantime? Something called the Industrial Revolution, which permitted food processing at a huge scale. For the sake of profit, the food has lower quality and also lower price than organic food, and guess what? It even causes addiction. It somehow makes you buy the same food, over and over again because you need more of it to cover your basic macronutrients needs.

Unfortunately, the food of today is focused more on caloric value than nutritional value, and the worst part is that we are too exposed to it. Finding organic food in urban areas is quite a difficult task, as pesticides are used on fruits, chemical fertilizers are used on vegetables and other legumes, and animals are being fed concentrated food before being slaughtered. This is how a chicken grows so fast, but this affects also other animals. All of these factors influence the quality of our food and may lead to several diseases, especially related to high blood sugar levels. Diabetes was not a very common disease a few centuries ago, but now it's amongst the most spread diseases worldwide. Heart, kidney, or liver diseases are very common, but also neurodegenerative diseases like Alzheimer's or Parkinson's disease are becoming more and more "popular." How we can reverse all of these and put a stop to it? Is medication a solution? Medication is not designed to cure, but instead, it was designed to make the disease a bit more pleasant by masking the symptoms. In a positive scenario, it can only stimulate the body to overcome the disease. The body heals itself, so why use a medicine, especially when it comes to common conditions and diseases like high blood sugar and insulin, heart, kidney, and liver diseases.

Autophagy is the answer to all these problems, and in this book, you can learn how you can activate it and what benefits it has. In this book, you will discover different methods on how to induce or activate autophagy. Although some of them may sound discouraging, you can find in here important tips on how to practice these methods, how to maximize their effects and of course, the benefits of each method. You can discover important information about Intermittent Fasting, Ketosis, HIIT, and Protein Fast. The cure for all of the diseases mentioned above is within your grasp, and the best part is that you don't have to pay serious cash for medicine. After reading this book, you will think again before buying medicine for such diseases and therefore save a lot of money. Autophagy is not holistic or "voodoo" medicine, it is something real, something that won the Nobel prize a few years ago, so it's a practice that you should take it very seriously. There are plenty of reasons why you should consider getting your body into autophagy mode, and you can find all of them if you read the chapters of this book. There is only one more thing left to say. Enjoy your reading!

Part One - Autophagy

History of Autophagy

The term "Autophagy" can trace its origins in the Greek words "phagy" (which happens to mean eat) and "auto" (which obviously means self). However, this doesn't mean that it was studied in Ancient Greece. Putting them together, we can conclude that autophagy is basically self-eating, but a more detailed definition can be seen in the sub-chapter below. The first studies related to this field were done in the late 1950s, but only after the 1990s, the progress was more significant. This concept is "a conserved cellular pathway that controls protein and organelle degradation, and has essential roles in survival, development, and homeostasis. Autophagy is also integral to human health and is involved in physiology, development, lifespan, and a wide range of diseases, including cancer, neurodegeneration, and microbial infection."[i]

This concept was born when a few scientists studied the membrane-bound compartments in the kidneys of small lab animals like mice. Clark and Novikoff first noticed mitochondria from mouse kidneys, when they studied the membrane-bound compartments, which also include lysosomal enzymes. Porter and Ashford discovered later endoplasmic reticulum and semi-digested mitochondria in the membrane-bound vesicles of rat's hepatocytes which were exposed to glucagon, but Essner and Novikoff discovered lysosomal hydrolases in the same bodies. At the Ciba Foundation symposium on lysosomes in 1963, a scientist called de Duve founded the discipline in which he emphasized the "autophagy" concept as describing the existence of a single or double-membrane vesicle with parts of organelles and cytoplasm in a different state of disintegration. He named "autophagosomes" the sequestering vesicles and claim that they occur in normal cells and are related to lysosomes. There are still a few controversies when it comes to the origin of membranes around the autophagosome, and de Duve thinks that they come from preformed membranes, like endoplasmic reticulum.

Apparently, cellular autophagy can be noticed in the normal liver cells of rats, and it even increases in the livers of starving animals. It was in 1967 when Deter and de Duve have advised that autophagy is induced by glucagon. Just ten years later, Pfeifer had proven that insulin prevents autophagy. Studies conducted by Schworer and Mortimore proved that amino acids prevent autophagy in rat liver cells. "Subsequently, Seglen and Gordon carried out the first biochemical analysis of autophagy and identified the pharmacological reagent 3-methyladenine as an autophagy inhibitor; they also provided the first evidence that protein kinases and phosphatases can regulate autophagy".[ii]

The period between the 1950s and 1980s is marked by morphological analyses in the studies of autophagy. de Duve suggested in the 1960s that most of the living cells (probably all of them) have to use a mechanism for digestion and bulk separation of cytoplasm in the lysosome, but he also suggested the demand of a proteolytic mechanism which has to be selective and to act on atypical organelles or cellular proteins. It was in 1973 when Weibel and Bolender demonstrated that the endoplasmic reticulum could be consumed by autophagy. Lockskin and Beaulaton pointed out that during insect metamorphosis, mitochondria are cleared selectively (1977). Another milestone in the study of autophagy is marked by the year 1983 when Veenhuis discovered that autophagy degrades selectively superfluous peroxisomes in the *Hansenula polymorpha* yeast. In the late 1980s,

Lemasters proved that the burst of autophagy could be caused by amendments in the mitochondrial membrane.

The golden age of autophagy had begun in the early 1990s. It was also called the Genetical or Molecular Era. The studies from this period were focused on selective and nonselective autophagy in yeast. "In 1992, Ohsumi and colleagues described the presence of "autophagic bodies" in the vacuole (the analog of the lysosome) of protease-deficient *Saccharomyces cerevisiae* devoid of nutrients—the first morphological characterization of nonselective autophagy in yeast."[iii] However, that was not all, as scientists like Klionsky and Dunn also conducted a few very important studies related to autophagy. "In the same issue of the *Journal of Cell Biology*, Klionsky et al. described the import of aminopeptidase I into the vacuole of *Saccharomyces cerevisaie*—the first characterization of selective autophagy in yeast. Shortly thereafter, Dunn and colleagues described a form of selective autophagy in the methylotrophic yeasts, *Pichia pastoris* and *Hansenula polymorpha*, involving the selective degradation of peroxisomes in the vacuole."[iv]

These studies laid the groundwork to confine mutants in S. *cerevisiae* and to copy the genes cyphering the yeast autophagy process, which are referred to as autophagy-related genes (ATG). Other studies were conducted in methylotrophic yeasts. "Ohsumi's group (**22**) performed a genetic screen to isolate mutants that accumulate autophagic bodies in the vacuole and show decreased viability during nitrogen starvation (originally known as the *apg* mutants); Thumm et al. performed a genetic screen to isolate yeasts deficient in protein uptake for degradation in the vacuole (originally known as the *aut* mutants); and Klionsky's group performed a screen for mutants deficient in the delivery of a resident vacuolar hydrolase from the cytoplasm to the vacuole (originally known as the *cvt* mutants)."[v]

October 1996 marks a very important milestone in the study of autophagy because that's when the first yeast autophagy gene was reported by Dr. Ohsumi and his colleagues. This gene was "baptized" APG5 or ATG5. This was followed very shortly by the cloning of AUT1 (known today as ATG3) by the Thumm's group in February 1997. This gene encodes the E2-conjugating enzyme, which is also behind the change of the ubiquitin-like protein Atg8. "Mizushima et al. described a protein conjugation system in yeast, the Atg12–Atg5 system that requires a ubiquitin activating E1-like enzyme, Atg7, and in 1999, three additional groups reported in back-to-back papers the cloning and characterization of yeast *ATG7*. In 2000, Ichimura et al. reported that the Atg7 E1-like enzyme conjugates Atg8 to phosphatidylethanolamine, establishing a role for protein lipidation in membrane dynamics during autophagy."[vi]

After the year 2000, the researches (especially on *S. cerevisiae)* having biochemical, genetical and structural approaches continued to prove how autophagy works, but they also have emphasized a few extra components which are very important for different types of selective autophagy. All the progress related to the autophagy research were not left unnoticed, therefore, on October 3, 2016, Yoshinori Ohsumi was awarded the Nobel Prize in Physiology or Medicine, because of his "discoveries of the mechanisms for autophagy." This is how studies (from the 1990s) conducted on a simple organism, like the baker's yeast, practically helped Dr. Ohsumi to win the Nobel Prize.

What is Autophagy?

As mentioned in the previous sub-chapter, the term autophagy comes from the Greek notions "auto" (self) and "phagein" (to eat), so in a very basic explanation, it means to eat oneself. However, a more detailed definition shows us that autophagy is the mechanism of the body that disposes of old and old and damaged cells like proteins, organelles, and cell membranes, when the body doesn't have enough energy to maintain the old and damaged cell machinery (composed of all the cell types mentioned above). Autophagy is a process that recycles and degrades different cellular components, and it shouldn't be confused with apoptosis (although is similar), which is a process that schedules cell death. Apoptosis may sound a bit cruel, but just like an old car which is not functioning anymore, you have to get rid of old cells which are not functioning as they should be. The process disposes of the old cells, replacing them with new ones when those cells are not working as they did in the initial phase.

Autophagy is similar to apoptosis, it basically does the same thing, but this process is done at a subcellular level. If apoptosis is replacing the whole car, autophagy is replacing its parts. That's why it's responsible for the destruction of subcellular organelles, but also with rebuilding and replacing them with new ones. The lysosome organelle plays a crucial role in the autophagy process, as its enzymes are responsible for degrading the proteins from old subcellular components. This process, which activates at a subcellular level is enabled when the body is experiencing different types of metabolic stress like hypoxia, growth factor depletion, and nutrient deprivation. Every cell may dispose of subcellular parts and recycle them into new proteins or energy needed to survive. This is why the autophagy process can be regarded as a cellular housekeeper because it cleans the dead sub-cellular parts and replaces them with new ones. There are a few types of autophagy, including chaperone-mediated autophagy, macroautophagy, and microautophagy.

"Autophagy's main roles are:

- Remove defective proteins and organelles
- Prevent abnormal protein aggregate accumulation
- Remove intracellular pathogens."[vii]

When autophagy gets triggered, there are organelles from healthy cells, which tracks downs diseased or dead cells in order to consume them. This process is arbitrated by the *autophagosome,* an organelle which combines the lysosome and endosome to form a double membrane around the cell that's about to get eaten. The cell is getting dissolved and then converted into energy. There are still plenty of uncertainties when it comes to the origins of the autophagosome, but apparently is being formed when there are many ATG proteins at a site called "*pre-autophagosomal structure*" (PAS). There were notices a few similar structures located in the mammalian cells, but there aren't too many known details about the PAS.

Usually, autophagy gets activated by nutrient starvation:

- In yeast, different factors like starvation of nitrogen, auxotrophic amino acids, nucleic acid, carbon or even sulfate can trigger autophagy;

- In a plant cells environment, autophagy can also be activated by nitrogen and carbon starvation;

- At mammals, autophagy can occur in different degrees and also in various tissues. It can be noticed muscle, brain, liver, mitophagy in the Chaperone-Mediated Autophagy and mitochondria.

The reduction of amino acids can signal autophagy activation. However, this can also depend on the amino acids and cell types, as amino acid metabolism can be different among tissues;

- The endocrine system, especially the insulin, also regulates autophagy. By increasing the blood sugar and warning about the presence of the nutrients, insulin crushes liver autophagy. The counterpart of insulin (glucagon), releases the glycogen from the liver to be burned for energy, and this enhances autophagy.

Autophagy should be regarded as a catabolic pathway that determines you to destroy old cells. Even though autophagy leads to protein breakdown, it's still required for muscle homeostasis. In the case of poor functioning autophagy, your body would have to seriously maintain lean tissue. This process helps your body to handle easier atrophy and catabolism by promoting protein austerity. An inadequate or weakened state of autophagy can lead to muscle wasting and aging. Also, excessive or defective autophagy can contribute to loss of lean tissue and muscle disorders. The ways to keep cells alive and to build new tissues are through insulin and mTOR (which are both anabolic). That's why bodybuilders and other athletes focus on having an anabolic lifestyle in order to prevent muscle catabolism. They consume protein supplements, and various amino acids to grow their muscles. One way to suppress autophagy is to have nutrients and access to energy constantly. When you have a constant flow of macronutrients, all of these substances are not used for energy, and this leads to less responsive cells. In order to assimilate and absorb the nutrients, you will need to mildly stare yourself, because you will be more sensitive when it comes to these nutrients and your cells will start to become more responsive. Autophagy is vital when it comes to supporting the plasticity of the skeletal muscle as a reply to endurance exercise. For autophagy to be enabled during exercise, AMPK (adenosine monophosphate-activated protein kinase) needs to be triggered also. AMPK is an enzyme that is very important to the homeostasis of cellular energy, by activating the uptake of fatty acid and glucose (and oxidation too) when the cellular energy is low. Also, it adjusts the breakdown pathways and protein synthesis. AMPK gets activated when the body is experiencing tough exercise, nutrient deprivation, and energy stress. The best time to exercise is when the body is in a fasted state because there are higher levels of LC3B-II compared to the fed state. This fact also shows that there is a better autophagic response when the exercise is done in a fasted state. In this case, the body goes straight for the fat tissue when it comes to the energy source, instead of burning the nutrients from the food you just had. AMPK contributes to better oxidation of the fatty acid and also enhances the glycolysis flux, whilst preventing the synthesis of cholesterol, fatty acid, and gluconeogenesis.

"In addition, AMPK has been recently shown to be a critical regulator of skeletal muscle protein turnover. Protein turnover is the balance between protein build up and protein breakdown over the course of the day.

- If your protein synthesis exceeds the amount protein's being broken down, then you're in a more anabolic state.

- If you're breaking down more than synthesizing, then you'll be more catabolic. Or autophagic."[viii]

The human body oscillates between anabolism and catabolism, both of these states are important for a healthy life, as you want to grow and repair your vital muscles and organs, but you also want to get rid of the metabolic debris and old cells. If you are wondering when autophagy happens, there is no exact answer, as it happens in different degrees most times (if not all the times). AMPK was just mentioned, but to understand autophagy, you also need to understand mTOR (which will be detailed in the sub-chapter below). By suppressing the insulin and mTOR, the chances of getting the autophagy increase in a different degree. Lower liver glycogen and blood glucose indicate the energy deficit in the body. As the energy level is getting lower, the body activates the metabolic pathways linked with burning fat tissue for fuel. This leads to higher ketones level in the blood, so a ketotic state of the body. Keeping insulin and blood glucose low helps with maintaining autophagy when the levels of fatty acids and endogenous ketones are getting higher. Usually, autophagy and ketosis are going "hand-in-hand," but there are some situations when you can be in a ketosis state without triggering autophagy, or the other way around, to induce autophagy without being in the ketosis state. How is this possible? Well, everything comes down to mTOR and nutrient signaling. Insulin is negatively influenced by exogenous ketones and fats, but they can still activate mTOR if consumed in large amounts in wrong circumstances. You can notice amounts of autophagy when fasting for 24 hours after a diet which is very rich in carbs. However, to make sure you experience the full benefits of autophagy, you will have to fast for at least 48 hours, giving plenty of time for the immune system and stem cells to work their "magic." Some autophagy specialists like Siim Land would recommend 3-5 days fast to be done 2-3 times per year. These procedures will help you burn a lot of the body fat quite easily, but will also encourage the recycling of weak cells, which might cause you some issues. If you have a lifestyle with 3 main meals per day, with plenty of snack and consumption of food rich in carbs and fats, you may experience a situation of excessive overconsumption which will never lead to autophagy and recycling old cells. You are basically keeping the body overfed and not leaving it to clean itself.

"Even people who eat "clean foods" but don't go through nutrient starvation may potentially be walking trash cans. There are many other sources of toxins and inflammation all of us get exposed to starting from air pollution, water, GMOs, plastics, heavy metals, and who knows what else. What looks good on the outside doesn't mean that everything is okay on the inside. Having your autophagy pathways live and active is even more important for living in the modern world."[ix]

What is mTOR, How It Affects the Autophagy and How to Balance It?

In order to experience cellular growth, you will need lipids, amino acids, and most of all, significant amounts of energy. The body monitors and adjusts the cells' energy and the nutrient status in order to keep homeostasis. mTOR stands for the mammalian target of rapamycin and is one of the main mechanisms responsible for the anabolic state of the body and for its growth. This mechanism is triggered by the same growth factors and nutrients responsible for activating muscle protein synthesis (MPS), and it's linked to hypertrophy, which is new cells and tissue development. mTOR can affect hypertrophy at least indirectly, as it connects to cellular growth and protein synthesis using plenty of pathways. Also, there are 2 mTOR complexes:

mTORC1 and mTORC2. Both of these complexes can encourage the immune system, muscle building, angiogenesis, protein synthesis, DNA repair, proliferation, and of course, cell growth.

- mTORC1 regulates protein synthesis. as it acts as a nutrient sensor. It's controlled by glucose, phosphatidic acid, ATP (energy molecules) oxygen levels, oxidative stress, mechanical stimuli, amino acids, growth factors, and insulin. mTORC1 is the most important factor when it comes to the protein synthesis of skeletal muscle.

- mTORC2 controls the actin cytoskeleton, which represents some long chains of proteins located in the cytoplasm of eukaryotic cells.

This is how mTOR works:

- your body directs energy to the right places when it senses too much energy in the system;

- amino acids, proteins, IGF-1 (growth factor) and insulin trigger the mTOR complexes;

- The tyrosine kinase receptors include the IGF-1 Receptor and also the Insulin Receptor. Tyrosine is considered an amino acid. Enabling these receptors can also lead to the phosphorylation of IRS (insulin substrate receptor);

- "IRS activates a protein called phosphatidylinositol-3-kinase (PI3K) which further phosphorylates inositol phospholipids like PIP3. PIP3 interacts with proteins PDK1 and Akt.

- Akt is thought to be one of the main upstream regulators of mTOR. Akt is a family of proteins that comprise of Akt1, Akt2, and Akt3. Akt1-2 are expressed in skeletal muscle while Akt3 is not."[x]

- When there is a plethora of nutrients around, mTORC1 pairs with ULK1, which is a kinase capable of activating autophagy and suppresses the formation of the autophagosomes which can trigger autophagy. At that point when the energy gets drained, mTORC1 turns inactive and it self-discharges from the ULK1 complex, setting free the formation of autophagosomes.

A growth factor which is known to constrain muscle growth by restraining hypertrophy is myostatin. In simple words, this growth factor it's an attempt to preserve energy from an evolutionary point of view by trying not to build too much muscle. It can lower the protein synthesis and completely stop the muscle cell copying process. ULK1, AMPK, and mTORC1 can form a vital trinity to maintain nutrient homeostasis and energy, also known as The Kinase Triad.

There seems to be an evolutionary path between anabolism and catabolism, but also between growth and repair. Anabolism is linked with growth, as an anabolic organism can grow very fast, but it can also speed up the biological clock in such a way that it can lead to oxidative stress of the mitochondria or to organs working very hard. Growing fast means also aging faster. The catabolism state favors cells degrading at a fast pace, faster than your body can repair. This situation can eventually damage important cells or other processed in your body. In such a case, you will not live very long due to physical deterioration. Clearly, you need both anabolism and catabolism for better health and longevity. The first one is very good for your bone structure and muscle mass, whilst the second one is vital for controlling your fuel sources and preventing unnecessary loss of energy. Somehow, you need to find a way to balance them.

"Basically, the expression of mTOR and its precursors is the most important signaling pathway in your body because mTOR will tell the body what's its energy status. If your physiology is in a state of nutrient deprivation and starvation, your body recognizes that it's not the best time to grow."[xi] mTOR usually inclines the balance towards excessive anabolism, so stimulating it during the day it's something you definitely want to avoid. In order to live longer, the body will need to recycle its own cells for most of the time, and mTOR should be triggered just for a short time to have a massive effect. Trying a nutrient dense very consistent diet, which can stop mTOR for most of the time, but can activate it just for muscle building. According to Ron Rosedale, MD, an anti-aging expert who is concerned about too much protein intake because of mTOR: "Health and lifespan are determined by the proportion of fat versus sugar people burn throughout their lifetime. The more fat that one burns as fuel, the healthier the person will be, and the more likely they will live a long time. The more sugar a person burns, the more disease ridden and the shorter a lifespan a person is likely to have."[xii]

Getting into the ketosis state and then into autophagy, may not be enough to live longer, as there are some cancers and tumors that are favored by ketone bodies. Regulating your metabolic pathway and being fully aware of the direction you are going with your diet plan can be the solution in this case. Intermittent Fasting it's very important for life extension (any diet without IF doesn't have an anti-aging effect) as well for balancing mTOR using autophagy. Protein restriction can't have the same positive effects as true fast, just like the keto diet may maintain the glycogen and insulin level low, but in order to experience the full-scale benefits of autophagy, you will need some periods with an energy deficit. Autophagy means that your cells are eating themselves and making them reborn. It is a continuous cycle, and the more active this cycle is, the longer you will live.

Why is Autophagy Important and What Are Its Benefits?

As previously mentioned, autophagy acts as a cellular housekeeper, whose main roles are to remove intracellular pathogens, defective organelles, and proteins and also to avoid the accumulation of abnormal proteins. Autophagy can help prevent some aging-related diseases like neurodegenerative diseases (Parkinson's), Alzheimer's disease, cancer, or atherosclerosis. Only by using this argument, you can establish that autophagy is good for your body. "Autophagy has many anti-aging benefits because it helps destroy and reuse damaged components occurring in vacuoles (spaces) within cells. In other words, the autophagy process basically works by using waste produced inside cells to create new "building materials" that aid in repair and regeneration."[xiii]

By now, there is no doubt that autophagy plays a major role in "cleaning up" the body and protecting it from the negative effects of stress. Autophagy studies are still on an incipient phase, but the benefits of it we know already are:

- builds molecular blocks and energizes cells;

- recycles aggregates, organelles, and damaged proteins;

- regulates the functions of the cells of mitochondria, which can play an important role in the producing energy process, but can be harmed by factors like oxidative stress;

- clears peroxisomes and damaged endoplasmic reticulum;

- defends the nervous system and favors the growth of nerve and brain cells. Although there may be some doubts, autophagy may play a significant role in improving the neuroplasticity, brain structure, and cognitive function;

- protects against heart diseases and encourages the growth of heart cells;

- eliminates the intracellular pathogens and improves the immune system;

- protects the body from toxic proteins that may contribute to amyloid diseases;

- defends the DNA's stability;

- prevents necrosis (damage to healthy organs and tissues);

- can potentially fight against neurodegenerative diseases, cancer, and other illnesses.

As studies have shown (first studies were conducted on mice and rats), autophagy can occur to different living organisms besides humans. It can be noticed at other mammals, plants, mold, yeast, flies or worms. So far, there were discovered at least 32 various autophagy-related genes (Atg). For plenty of species, autophagy is a response to stress and starvation (which can be induced through fasting or nutrient deprivation). As the autophagy process can play an important role in preventing or fighting against cancer, neurodegenerative diseases, or other diseases, you need to understand how this is possible. Below you can find how autophagy acts when it comes to cancer or Parkinson disease.

Can autophagy suppress tumors?

When it comes to cancer, it has become a generally accepted idea that autophagy can prevent tumor initiation. But how is this possible? If you think about it, it makes sense because autophagy can block the growth and enhance the breakdown of the proteins. In cancer cells, there is usually a lower level of basal autophagy, compared to other normal cells. Just to prove the point (autophagy's effect on cancer), there are plenty of studies of the tumor-suppressor genes and oncogenes which are tightly linked to autophagy. Only when you think of the PTEN tumor-suppressor gene, it has been shown that it blocks PI3K/Akt, and therefore activates autophagy. The mutations of this gene are usually discovered in cancer, leading to a decreased autophagy and enhanced risk of cancer. Although it appears that the autophagy state can be the opposite of the increased risk of cancer state, it's not a general rule. In the unfortunate situation when cancer progresses, there is nothing that autophagy can do to it to reverse it. On the contrary, it can contribute to cancer survival, exactly how it helps all cells to survive in a stressful habitat. When the body experiences nutrient deprivation, autophagy wants to use the amino acids from proteins as energy. In the event of fast-growing cancer, enhanced autophagy can help it spread because it provides the required energy and deals with the stress.

Autophagy's effect on Neurodegenerative Diseases like Parkinson Disease, Alzheimer Disease, and Huntington's chorea

All of these diseases and conditions manifest in a different way, but they all have something in common, a pathologic similarity. In the case of Alzheimer's humans can experience memory loss and other cognitive modifications, with Parkinson's there is resting tremor and loss of voluntary movement and when it comes to Huntington's chorea, there are some involuntary movements noticed.

However, the pathologic similarity in all these cases is the excessive accumulation of proteins inside neurons causing dysfunction and eventually disease. "Thus, failure of protein degradation pathways may play a very important role in preventing these diseases. However, the exact role of autophagy in these diseases is still yet to be defined. Further, growing research also implicates mitochondrial dysfunction as a key pathway in the development of neurodegenerative diseases."[xiv]

Conducting studies on humans is something very difficult to do as there are many intersecting pathways. However, taking drugs can provide clear evidence because one pathway can be modified at a time. mTOR acts as a nutrient sensor, especially for amino acid, and when mTOR is blocked, autophagy is triggered. When there are no nutrients to be consumed, mTOR decreases, and autophagy increases. Different mTOR inhibitors like everolimus and rapamycin are able to block it, confusing the body and convincing it that there is nutrient deprivation. This scenario enhances autophagy. Drugs taken for these diseases have immune-suppressing consequences in transplant medicine. Although most immune-suppressing drugs can enhance the risk of cancer, rapamycin is the exception. In some cases, mTOR inhibitors prove to have anticancer effects. A drug like Metformin, which is used for type 2 diabetes, can trigger autophagy, but through a different pathway than mTOR. Instead, it enhances AMPK, a molecule that shows how energized the cell is. High level of AMPK is linked with low energy levels in cells and helps to increase the autophagy. AMPK can feel the ADP/ATP ratio, so the energy level of the cell. When the level of this molecule is high, it influences, directly and indirectly, the activation of autophagy, but it also produces mitochondria.

Mitophagy is a process responsible for tracking down selectively dysfunctional or defective mitochondrion, which are the cellular powerhouses, the cell components that produce energy. When they are not working as they should, then mitophagy targets them to be destroyed. One of the mitophagy's regulators is PTEN, a tumor suppressor gene. This may not sound very good, but when mitophagy is enhanced, the new mitochondrion is stimulated to grow and develop. AMPK can favor the growth of both mitophagy and new mitochondrion, and this leads to swapping old mitochondrion with new ones. Metformin is the type of drug which can also have a positive impact on autophagy and AMPK, besides its impact on blood sugar.

If autophagy has such great results when it comes to preventing such diseases, what exactly is the relationship with the muscle mass? You might be inclined to think that nutrient deprivation will lead to muscle loss, as your body doesn't receive the necessary proteins to maintain the current muscles. If you do lose muscles during fasting, this is because autophagy gets inhibited. In order to maintain muscle mass, autophagy is required. Let's picture two different scenarios:

- when your body goes through a caloric restriction special diet, but for some reason, autophagy is blocked, you will end up in a semi-starvation state because your body doesn't switch to ketosis. This is the kind of situation which favors gluconeogenesis (the metabolic process that can create glucose from non-carb sources) and other severe stuff.

- let's say that autophagy gets activated if you are on a water fasting program or on fast mimicking. This situation will lead to the stimulation of the growth hormones, and thanks to it, your muscles will be preserved.

Autophagy can help preserve your muscle mass, if you don't consume any calories at all, instead of having just a few of them. Just a small bite of food can block the effect of autophagy, and the growth hormone is no longer being stimulated. "Even as little as 50 calories of 2-3 grams of leucine will stop autophagy and shift into a fed state. It's going to be better for fat loss, for muscle sparing and for longevity, to avoid all calories during your fasting window. That goes back to the idea of timing your calorie intake more in the post-workout scenario wherein you've reaped the benefits of fasting ketosis and are now prone to recover."[xv]

The most recommended way to be on a diet or a mild caloric deficit plan is ketosis because this phase will keep your lean tissue and will activate the fat burning process. There is no coincidence that your body enters the ketosis phase at the same time when it starts the fasted state. This is when the body switches the "fuel type" from glucose (mostly originated from carbs) to fats. In this phase, you will be only burning fats. Strangely, the longer you fast (with no calories at all), the higher the growth hormone is. However, muscles can't be preserved without exercising, so make sure you spent some time at the gym, you can also try jogging, cycling or swimming. Try an activity which will engage most muscles in your body.

Autophagy sounds like a "miracle agent" that can help the prevention of cancer, Alzheimer's Disease, Parkinson's Disease, Huntington's chorea, and other illnesses and conditions. However, these are some downsides to it, not just benefits. You can find below some negative consequences of autophagy. This process is also known as the autophagic flux, and it includes 3 different steps, "the formation of an autophagosome, fusion with lysosomes, and the degradation of the autophagosome."[xvi]

- Autophagy regulates immunity and inflammation by disposing of the inflammasome activators. When pathogens are removed by autophagy, the process is called xenophagy, which has plenty of immune-strengthening advantages. Although this may sound very good, a bacterium called Brucella can use autophagy to multiply themselves. This can lead to bacterial overgrowth (preventing the death of it when the bacteria should be extinct.

- It was discovered that an autophagy gene called ATG6/BECN1 concealing the Beclin1 protein could prevent tumors in cancer. However, this gene is not very effective when it comes to preventing tumors in cancer, and there are some situations when it can favor cancer because of the self-replicative process. Self-eating can favor tumor cell fitness as opposed to environmental stressors, so the tumor cells are more resilient when it comes to chemotherapy and starvation. The truth is that autophagy can't make any difference in cancer treatment, only in prevention.

- There are some doubts if autophagy stops or encourages programmed cell death or apoptosis. The result apparently depends on the cell type and stimulus. Stopping autophagy increases the bufalin pro-apoptotic effect on the gastric cancer cell. Bufalin is a medical toxin from China, which is very useful of suppressing tumor over endoplasmic reticulum stress. In this case, lower autophagy meant more cancer cell death due to the weakness of cancer cells. Apparently, with autophagy, cancer cells became stronger.

When put through nutrient deprivation, the malignant tumor cells may be prevented by autophagy from dying by suppressing apoptosis. So, not everything is fine with autophagy, as it has its disadvantages. Some pathogens and viruses are destroyed through autophagy, whilst others benefit from its mechanism and manage to multiply. Autophagy has different levels and acts differently in various tissues of the human body. It can't be the same in fat, muscle, liver, or brain. It doesn't have all the time positive effects on the tissues, but you do need positive autophagic impacts on the liver and the brain, but you don't want to experience the self-eating process on your muscles and lean tissue.

The entropy is a process responsible for the slow degradation and deterioration of the cells. You definitely want to avoid necrotic or dysfunctional apoptotic processes which can lead to a lesser and weakened state of your body. As a general rule of thumb, dispose of the bad cells (and replace them with new ones), but also keep the good ones, this is how autophagy should work.

Part Two – Inducing Autophagy

Ketosis

Many times, ketosis is associated with Intermittent Fasting, as it is a state which usually comes 12 hours after your last meal. At that point, the body starts to run on fats, so it switches the energy source from glucose to fats. To better understand ketosis, you will need to know better terms like carbohydrates, glucose, insulin, and of course, ketones.

Carbohydrates (also known as carbs) are a major macronutrient group which can be found in food types like bread, pasta, rice, potatoes, and grain. These are the main sources of carbs, but nowadays, everything processed has higher carb levels. The modern western diet, unfortunately, includes plenty of carbs. Carbohydrates are also known to be the main source of **glucose**, the default "fuel type" (energy) of the body. However, eating high amounts of carbs increases the blood sugar and insulin level, as the glucose is not consumed by the body, so it gets stored in the blood. A sedentary life correlated with high consumption of carbs can lead to serious consequences for the body. One major disease it can leave to is type 2 diabetes. Glucose is also known as dextrose, which is a simple sugar, very present in carbs. It is the primary energy source for the body, and in plenty of cases, it doesn't get fully consumed, as the body consumes too many carbs and even training doesn't fully use it, or it simply remains unconsumed (or used just in small amounts) due to a sedentary way of life. When glucose is not used, it gets stored into the blood, and therefore, it increases the blood sugar level. **Insulin** is released by the pancreas, and it is considered the main anabolic hormone of the body. Also, this hormone regulates the blood sugar level in your body, so it's vital in preventing a disease like diabetes. At some point, due to high carbs consumed, the glucose level is too high, so it massively gets stored into your blood. In some cases, this is too much for insulin to handle, so the body is in an insulin-resistant state. In this scenario, the body doesn't use insulin at all, although the body tends to produce more insulin than ever. This can be prevented from happening with a healthy diet and physical exercise. When the body is no longer receiving glucose, the ketones level from your body is increasing. **Ketones** are chemicals produced by your level, capable of breaking down fatty acids. This happens when the body goes into the fasted state when the body switches the fuel from glucose to fats.

Almost all the important terms were covered in the section below, but there is still one more - **ketosis**. This concept defines a metabolic state, during which the body consumes fats and uses ketones instead of glucose. "In ketosis, your body produces ketones at an accelerated rate. Ketones, or ketone bodies, are made by your liver from fat that you eat and your own body fat. The three ketone bodies are beta-hydroxybutyrate (BHB), acetoacetate, and acetone (although acetone is technically a breakdown product of acetoacetate)."[xvii]

Your liver is responsible for producing ketones, and it does its job even when the body is on a high carb diet. This happens overnight, during your sleep, but only in small amounts. When the insulin and glucose level decreases, that's when the liver can boost the production of ketones, so necessary to break down the fatty acids required for energy in this case. The level of ketones you have to reach, in order for your body to be considered in ketosis is debatable. Ketogenic diet researchers like Dr. Jeff Volek and Dr. Steve Phinney consider that the minimum level of BHB (the ketone level measured in the blood) in order for the body to reach ketosis has to be 0.5 mmol/L.[xviii]

Ketosis will not guarantee a fat loss, as a person can have high levels of ketones, but not to lose an ounce of fat, because he eats too much. However, this scenario is highly unlikely or very rare because overeating is not something that happens too often during a state of ketosis. Ketones are known for making you lose your appetite, but somehow people can find a way to eat more

Ketosis can be reached through Intermittent Fasting, or through a keto diet, but the last option can maintain the ketosis state for a longer period of time. This state is all about burning fats, so why not consume more fats? Is it harmful to the bodies? As it turns out, consuming fats can have a great positive impact on your body. The keto diet is based on fewer carbs and more fat, just to make sure your body burns the fat in an effective way. As indicated by more than 50 studies, the ketogenic diet (or short keto diet) can have plenty of benefits for performance, health and weight loss, being recommended and used by many doctors.[xix]

When it comes to losing excess body fat and even reversing type 2 diabetes, the keto diet proves to be very effective. As mentioned previously, the keto diet is an LCHF (low carbs high fat) diet. The modern-day standard "diet" includes too many carbs, and this is where keto diet can step in. It can replace most of the carbs with fats, inducing the metabolic state of ketosis. The body doesn't get enough glucose, so it needs to switch to a different energy source, and fat is the most "to hand" fuel type. However, to use the fat cells, you need something to break them down. The body already adapted, and increased the ketones levels, so now the body has the necessary tool to break down the fat cells and literally burn fat. Ketones release the energy stored in the fat cells in the entire body, so the body becomes very effective at burning fat. On top of that, the keto diet can significantly decrease the level of blood sugar and insulin, and on the other hand, it enhances the ketones level in your body. There are different types of keto diets, as you can see below:

- **Standard Ketogenic Diet** (SKD): involves very low consumption of carbs, moderate consumption of proteins, and high levels of fat. The percentage, in this case, is 75% fats, 20% protein, and only 5% carbs. You are probably worrying that such levels of fat will get you obese, but in order to avoid this from happening, you will need to seriously work out. This will not only burn the fats you are consuming, but it will also burn the fats you already have stored in your body;

- **Cyclical Ketogenic Diet** (CKD): if a "pure" keto diet is too harsh for you, then perhaps this one can work for you.

It combines days with higher carbs consumption with days with high fats and low carbs consumption. You can have 5 standard keto days and then 2 days with high-carb consumption;

- **Targeted Ketogenic Diet** (TKD): is the kind of meal plan which involves a higher-carb consumption around training;

- **High-Protein Ketogenic Diet**. This one is a slight adaptation of the standard ketogenic diet, as it involves a higher protein intake. The percentage, in this case, should be 60% fats, 35% protein, and just 5% carbs.

So far, studies were focused just on the standard keto diet and the high-protein ketogenic diet, but the targeted and cyclical diet are used more by athletes and bodybuilders. Your body will run on what you are feeding it, just like a car. Imagine that your body is a car, and since you are feeding it more fats, it will run on fat. Your fat tissue (or stored fat) is your "fuel tank" the body will attempt to empty (it will never succeed) in order to get more energy. This is how the keto diet works, it trains your body to run on fats, and therefore, in most cases, it will lead to increased levels of fat burned.

Since the recommended percentage of carbs is 5%, what exactly this means in numbers. The recommended amount of carbs should be under 50 grams, preferably under 20 grams. Getting the exact amount of macronutrients your meal has may not be the easiest task, but below you can find some interesting food types you can consume during a keto diet:

- Meat. The more processed the meat is, the more carbs it has. So, for a keto diet, you will need raw meat, and it the animal was fed with organic food or grass-fed even better. This food type is a great source of proteins (mostly) and fats. However, the keto diet doesn't consist of very high protein levels so you will need to limit the meat consumption, as the excess proteins will turn into glucose, which will prevent the ketosis state. Please try to avoid processed meats like sausages, meatballs and other types of processed foods, as they surely have carbs, and you will need to stick to just 5% carbs;

- Fish and seafood. They are very good for the keto diet, as they have a bit lower amount of proteins and if the fish is fatty like salmon, that's just great. Please avoid breading on fish, as they contain carbs;

- Eggs. This food type is recommended during a keto diet and can be consumed in any possible way (omelets, scrambled, boiled, and so on). Try to buy organic eggs, as they are the healthiest option;

- High-fat, or natural fat sauces. Lipids (also known as fats) should be the source of calories during a keto diet. Fat natural sauces can refer to coconut fat, or butter, but also other alternatives like olive oil, Bearnaise sauce or garlic butter. You don't have to avoid natural fat, but you will need to avoid other processed sauces, because guess what, they contain carbs;

- When it comes to vegetables, the general rule is to grow above ground; they can be green or leafy, fresh or frozen. The best keto veggies are zucchini, broccoli, avocado, cabbage, cauliflower. If you eat them in a salad, make sure you pour a consistent amount of olive oil. These kinds of vegetables can be a proper side dish and replacement for rice, potatoes, or pasta, which have plenty of carbs;

- High-fat dairy should not be missing

from a keto diet. Milk also contains carbs so you will need to avoid it, even if you are drinking a glass of it, consume it with cereals or just pour it into the coffee. You should have instead butter (especially for cooking, try to avoid consuming it spread on a slice of bread), high-fat cheese is very recommended, but yogurts with a higher concentration of fats should be consumed more moderately. Heavy cream can also be used for cooking. Try to avoid snacking on cheese, especially when there is no need for it (you are not hungry);

- Nuts. This food type should be consumed moderately, as you don't want to eat too much to feel satisfied. Some of the nuts like cashews have a higher concentration of carbs, so they should be avoided. Try instead pecan or macadamia nuts in smaller quantities;

- Berries should only be consumed in a

moderate amount on top of a dessert.

This is what it's recommended to eat during a keto diet, below you can take a look at what it's permitted to drink when being on such a diet.

- Water. There isn't a better option of drinks for any diet than water. It doesn't have any calories, and there isn't a known fluid or drink that can successfully replace water to cover all its functions. You can try it still, sparkling; you can add some ice cubes, slices of limes, lemon or cucumbers;

- Coffee. This type of drink is permitted within this kind of diet, but you will need to avoid sugar at any cost because this will introduce glucose in your body and therefore prevent the ketosis state. You can add instead a moderate amount of cream or milk. You can prepare yourself a "Bulletproof coffee" by adding butter or coconut oil to stir in the coffee.

If you notice that the weight loss process is not going as expected, you may need to eliminate the fat or cream from your coffee;

- Tea. This type of drink is highly recommended with the keto diet, so feel free to drink as many teas as you like, as long as they don't have any sugar. You can try Orange Pekoe, herbal, mint, green or black;

- Bone broth is also a drink you can try with this diet because it has plenty of electrolytes and nutrients, is hydrating and satisfying. For extra energy, you can add a bit of butter.

There are plenty of food types and drinks which are rich in carbs, and they all have to be avoided whilst being on a keto diet. Carbs can mostly come from sugar and starches, but there are also other food types with high carbs values. You can see them all below.

- Sugar. Is probably the most harmful ingredient you can consume. It can be found in plenty of sweets, soft drinks, fruit juices, candies, cookies, cakes, chocolate, ice cream, donuts, and breakfast cereals. There is no place for all these food types and drinks in a keto diet. Every time you purchase a product, you will have to check the label for the sugar level, and you can be amazed by how much sugar all the products from above have. Artificial sweeteners were designed to replace sugar, and they were meant to be less harmful, but they are still not recommended during a keto diet;

- Starch can be found different food types like bread, pasta, pastries, potatoes, French fries, potato chips, muesli, porridge, and rice. They all have to be avoided when being on a keto diet, as they have a high quantity of carbs. They are amongst the most common and popular food types, but they definitely have to be avoided when you are on a keto diet, and you want to lose weight. Some legumes, like lentils and beans, will have to be avoided also, as they are also rich in carbs. Since food types like rice, pasta, bread or porridge are very common and popular, the keto diet may include alternatives for all these products which comply with the rules of this diet (low on carbs, higher on fats);

- Beer is commonly known as liquid bread and is a drink that is very rich in carbs and will favor the quick absorption of its carbs. However, there are plenty of beer types all over the world, some of them are lower in carbohydrates;

- Very sweet fruits should also be avoided, as they contain the fruity type of sugar, is just like a natural candy;

- Margarine was intended to be a replacement for butter, and although some of these products have a higher content of omega-6 fat, they should be avoided. It's industrially produced (not from natural ingredients), tastes worse than butter and has little or no obvious benefits in terms of health.

Unfortunately, one of the most harmful addiction today is the one to carbs, as it affects most people nowadays. The devastating impact of carbs over your body can be the topic of plenty of books, articles, and even academic researches. However, when it comes to ketosis, you need to understand that this term is not exactly the same thing with the keto-adaption process. They are a bit different (although some people would disagree), as you can see below:

- Ketosis is the metabolic state with the appropriate blood sugar and ketone bodies level. "It's said that ketosis begins at 0.5mmol-s of blood ketones but having 0.3 mmol-s already is quite good. You can be in mild ketosis already after fasting for 24-hours, but it doesn't necessarily mean you're successfully using fat and ketones for fuel."[xx]

- On the other hand, keto-adaptation is the process responsible for making your body to use ketones and fat as the primary fuel type. Therefore, you don't have to depend any longer on glucose, and you can burn your own stored fat or the fats you are eating.

This process is not an exact science, so you don't know exactly when it has started. There are a few signs which might indicate that you switched to the fat-burning process. You will need to understand that everyone has the keto-adaptation process going on to some extent.

- when you consume not enough calories, you will definitely lose some fat;

- if your diet includes eggs and bacon, the body will get some energy form it;

- no matter of the activity you are doing, whether you are jogging or just walking, you will burn fat.

"The problem is that when you're not that well keto-adapted, and you're causing metabolic stress to your body through caloric restriction or exercising on an empty glycogen tank, then you're producing some ketones but your body isn't that efficient at using fat for fuel, you'll also start converting some of your muscle tissue into glucose through gluconeogenesis."[xxi]

The keto-adaption process is the only one that can establish how much fat you will be able to burn and also how much protein you will compensate.

- Being on a diet which is rich and carbs and proteins, but low on fats will determine glucose addiction and will cause frequent eating. It's the same issue with a diet rich in carbs and fructose because it encourages frequent eating to prevent anabolism;

- Trying the paleo approach with slightly lower levels of carbs transforms your body into an organism like a "hybrid car." Around 30-50% of your caloric intake can trace their origins from carbs, which may encourage the fat burning process, but after you burn the glucose first because you are still consuming more of it;

- Obviously, the ideal keto diet is the low carbs high-fat one. This type of diet encourages the keto-adaptation process, as it keeps you in the ketosis state, whilst your body is using ketones to break down fats, and therefore extracting the energy from the fat tissue (which has now become the primary energy source).

The main purpose of the keto diet should be the keto-adaptation process, not necessarily the ketosis nutritional state. In order to induce the keto-adaptation process, you will need to follow some steps. Below you can find all the necessary steps for this process:

1. Carb Restriction means literally cutting down on carbs using a ketogenic diet and therefore removing most of the carbs (even all of them) from your diet. You can eat fatty meat, eggs, fish and leafy vegetables;

2. Keto Flu Period is the period when you feel tired and exhausted, mostly because ketones are not used yet efficiently to break down the fatty cells and release the energy in the body. The brain will eventually adapt and will learn how to use the ketones to produce energy, but until then, you will experience the keto flu period. It may take from a few days to a few weeks to overcome this "flu,"

depending on how sensitive you are;

3. Getting Familiar to Ketones. After the keto flu period, you will start to feel better and to have increased energy levels, just by eating the standard keto diet. Intermittent Fasting can rush this process, but you will have to be careful not to starve yourself. This phase may last between 2 weeks to a few months, but in this case, the longer you are in this phase, the better;

4. Fat Burning Mode. Once you have recovered your energy after the keto flu period and the ketones are working properly, your body is officially in the fat burning mode. You will notice better performance, visible fat loss, but also faster period of recovery after workouts, decreased hunger, better mental clarity, less fatigue and longer time to exhaustion;

5. Keto Adaptation is when your body runs smoothly on body fat and the fat you consume, without craving for carbs to feel energized or to perform at optimal levels. Ketones are very active, they burn the fat cells, leading to less hunger;

6. Flexible Metabolism. At this point, you can also fuel your body with carbs (temporarily) and still be in the ketosis nutritional state. One of the most important goals of the keto-adaptation process is to avoid addiction to ketones or carbs and to consume or use both of them in different situations.

Ketosis has plenty of benefits for the body and for your health. Just think about it, a keto diet restricts the carbs consumption, which is the source of so many troubles for your body. Since there are so many diseases known to man caused by the food we eat, it's not an exaggeration to say that carbs are responsible for so many of these diseases. Ketones play a major role in reducing inflammation and oxidative stress, the roots for so many chronic diseases.

Some of the most important benefits of the ketosis state are:

a. Better control over your appetite. A good thing noticed by most of the people being in the ketosis state is that they don't experience hunger all the time. Researches have shown that ketosis inhibits appetite, as the consumption of carbs makes the body craving for more. As carbs are associated with glucose, which is a kind of energy source for the body, they are no longer needed in the keto diet, as the glucose gets stored in the blood, increasing the blood sugar and the insulin level;

b. Your body can lose weight. The most useful macronutrients are proteins and fats. To induce ketosis and to make sure the body runs on fats, you will need to consume mostly fats, less protein, and minimum amounts or none at all carbs. By doing this, the body will burn the fat reserves it has, and the fats provided by the keto diet. As mentioned above, the keto diet inhibits the appetite, but it also lowers the insulin level, whilst the ketones bodies are multiplying. This can only lead to increased fat burning, and therefore, weight loss.

c. Prediabetes and diabetes reversal. Ketosis regulates the blood sugar and also the insulin response because glucose levels are significantly lower. For people suffering from prediabetes and diabetes, this can lead to less (and even none) diabetes medication;

d. Better athletic performance. Since the ketosis state encourages fat burning, this will make the body stronger, more agile, and also faster. So, it's fair to say that it helps to improve athletic performance;

e. "Seizure management: Maintaining ketosis with the classical ketogenic diet or less stringent modified Atkins diet (MAD) has been proven effective for controlling epilepsy in both children and adults who don't respond to anti-seizure medication."[xxii]

When it comes to side effects of ketosis and the keto diet, the keto flu period (described at the keto-adaptation process) seems to be the main disadvantage. Some of the cures may include more water and salt, less physical activity, more fat in your diet and a slower decrease of the carb intake. Other side effects of ketosis are (although arguably) kidney damage, muscle loss, vitamin deficiency, and constipation. Some of these side effects will happen anyway, and some of them can be avoided by doing the keto diet properly.

As you will be depriving the body of carbs (almost entirely), it will increase the levels of ketones, the tool of extracting energy from the fat reserves. In fact, ketones can have plenty of protective effects. There are a few studies which indicate that ketosis can lead to starvation-induced autophagy, a state with neuroprotective functions.

Many bodybuilders or nutritionists would agree that switching to fasting can improve the fat burning process and also there are higher chances of preventing something like muscle loss, as the growth hormone reaches a very high level during fasting. However, more details related to fasting, how it works, how you can practice it, and what are its benefits, can be found in the sub-chapter below.

Fasting

Usually, the concept of Intermittent Fasting is tightly linked with autophagy, and to an extent, they are intertwined. Intermittent Fasting (also known as IF) is a process of self-discipline, during which you allow the body to use fat tissue as energy sources. Since fasting literally means not to eat and Intermittent Fasting means eating just in a very limited period of time, and the rest of the time you can only drink water, it's really no wonder that the body goes through a nutrient deprivation phase. Autophagy usually gets triggered after 24-48 hours of fasting. Intermittent Fasting was the first diet tried by humans, although this was done involuntarily. It has to be regarded as a procedure which has plenty of benefits for your body, in terms of health and well-being, but it shouldn't be regarded as a process to lose weight. Instead, it prepares the body for weight loss, as it needs to be associated with physical exercise for the fat burn process. In plain words, fasting means refraining yourself from consuming food for a period of time. Depending on the type of fast you want to try, the fast period can vary from 16, 18, 20, 24 hours, or even more. Unlike any other diet, fasting doesn't involve any special food requirements; you can eat what you normally eat, but within a certain period of time. From all the major nutrients we consume during a day, the highest percentage is represented by carbohydrates. They provide large amounts of glucose, which in this initial state is the body's default fuel or the primary energy source.

Without any doubt, Intermittent Fasting switches the energy source from glucose to fat tissue. Once the glucose is already consumed, as you are no longer eating to get more carbs and glucose, the body will search for another source of energy, and the fat tissue is a very good alternative when it comes to energy. The fast state is when the body runs out of glucose to use for energy. It is said that the body enters the fast state 12 hours from the last meal. From that point, the body runs on fats, so that's the best time to exercise and burn fat.

History of Fasting

Intermittent Fasting was the first diet tried by humans, although this was done involuntarily. In the prehistoric days, humans were relying on hunting, fishing, or just picking fruits to feed. Food was not available at every moment, so they literally had to starve before eating again. Fasting was more of a way of life, an involuntary diet caused by limited food availability. If today fasting can mean skipping breakfast on a regular basis, back then it meant something else completely. There was no certainty when the next meal would be, as weather conditions played a significant role in the probability of feeding. If the weather was favorable, humans could easily go hunting or fishing or picking fruits (if there were available). The prey was not guaranteed, and humans were sometimes required to travel extensively in search for it. It can be said that fasting made the humans stronger, faster, and more agile. It was the process that adapted their bodies to the surrounding environment. The prehistoric humans were consuming high-quality food, as the food was natural, and it had proper nutritional value. When humans discovered agriculture, daily meals were more diversified, and the percentage of meat started to decrease. However, during winter seasons, humans were still experiencing starvation, as they didn't know how to preserve food for the cold season. This season also meant a fasting period, as humans were required to return to old habits like hunting and fishing, in order to make sure they have enough food for the winter. As civilizations were flourishing all over the world, and humans were building proper shelters, the first cities and castles appeared. This form of organization also included some storage spaces, where people can put the grains and crops for the winter and consume them during the cold season. People were starting to forget about the lack of food, as it started to become available and abundant. There was no longer uncertainty when it came to the time of the next meal, (unless they were very poor), and people were starting to forget about fasting. Only religion kept the memory of fasting alive, and even today, fasting is practiced in various religions throughout the globe, like Islam, Judaism, or Christianity. The quality of the food was still very good, as most of the food was in a natural state. However, the industrial was about to change that, as it didn't just mean technological progress in terms of manufacturing, it also marked the birth of food processing. Slowly, the percentage of processed food started to increase, until it reached the level from today. There is no surprise that the majority of the food we consume today is processed, as natural food is becoming scarce and very difficult to find, especially for people living in an urban environment. It looks like more than 70% of the diseases known today are caused by the food we eat, and since we consume too much processed food, rich in carbs, this led to the conclusion that processed food can do serious damages to your health. According to religion, fasting is a way to cleanse your body and to achieve penitence. Although it's mostly practiced for religious purposes, this procedure is becoming more popular, as recent studies have shown the positive impact it can have on health. Nutritionists and other fitness enthusiasts now recommend Intermittent Fasting for all the benefits it can have on your body, health, and general well-being.

How to Practice Intermittent Fasting

IF can be regarded as a weight loss strategy, but above all, it's a very healthy lifestyle because it comes with plenty of benefits for your health. It trains the body to be more self-protective and efficient, whilst being familiarized with the modern times we are living in. This procedure usually divides the day or certain of time into eating period and fasting period, which are not quite exactly the same with the fed and fast state. Some of the specialists would agree that there are 5-6 different phases of Intermittent Fasting.

- 12 hours after the last meal, the body enters the fast state, but it also enters into a metabolic state named ketosis. During this state, the body starts to use fat cells as energy by switching from glucose to fats. In other words, this is the time when the body starts to run on fats and to burn fat.

- the second phase is the fat-burning mode, which is achieved after 18 hours. In this phase, the body generates copious amounts of ketones. The blood ketones levels are significantly higher than the normal values. Ketones play the role of signaling molecules which can inform "your body to ramp up stress-busting pathways that reduce inflammation and repair damaged DNA for example."[xxiii]

- according to some nutritionists, after 24 hours autophagy starts. This is the process of recycling and replacing old cell types or misfolded proteins associated with Alzheimer's or other illnesses.

- 48 hours after your last meal, the growth hormone level is absolutely huge, as it literally is 5 times bigger than it was at the beginning of the fasting period. Surprisingly, the lack of calories, proteins, and carbs lead to this situation so this can be a piece of very useful information for bodybuilders.

- by 54 hours, the insulin level is at its

lowest level since the beginning of the fast period, so your body is already becoming a lot more insulin sensitive.

- 72 hours after your last meal, the body is destroying old immune cells, and it develops new ones.

Although there aren't such requirements, choosing the right types of food can make fasting more effective. That's why people should avoid any type of food with little to nothing nutritional value, junk-food especially. Cutting down on carbs should be a high priority when it comes to choosing your food, as this can help the fasting process when it comes to burning fats. That's why some nutritionists would recommend an LCHF (low carbs high fats) diet because it favors the fat loss process, as you consume fewer carbs (the main source of glucose) and you eat more fats, and therefore you set the organism to use fats as the "default fuel."

If you don't have any medical condition, then you should definitely try Intermittent Fasting. You can choose from one of the most popular fasting programs you can find below and find out which one best suit your needs.

One of the best options out there, when it comes to IF programs are the **Leangains method**, or the 16/8 hour fast. This method is very popular amongst bodybuilders and other athletes, as this program favors the fat burning process. The program was developed by Mark Berkhan, and it consists of dividing the day into 2 different periods: the feeding window which should last no longer than 8 hours and the fasting window which should last 16 hours. You have to distinguish right from the start what is the difference between the fast state and fasting window. The last one is the period of time in which you are not eating (so not consuming any calories at all), whilst the fast state is when the body starts to consume fat as energy fuel after the glucose is no longer available. The fast state starts approximately 12 hours after the last meal, and that's when you need to work out, as it's the optimal time to burn fat. Fasting each day can have very good results for the fat burning process. 16 hours each day should be more than enough for the body to use the fat reserves as fuel. The default energy source is glucose, mostly obtained from carbs. However, when the body enters the fasted state, the moment marks the change of energy source from glucose to fat. Even if there aren't specific meal requirements, in order for the Leangains method to work even better, you need to eat healthily. Here are some rules you need to follow in order to maximize the effects of the Leangains method:

- Protein boosts should be a priority with most meals (when possible);

- The workout should be associated with this plan, as fasting works better with it;

- If you plan to eat plenty of carbs, you

should have them in the training days, whilst during those days when you are not training, you should focus on low carbs meals;

- You can have consistent meals during the feeding period (don't exaggerate though), and absolutely nothing to eat during the fasting period. Try to avoid any snacks during this period, as the only thing you should be putting in your mouth is water;

- The most consistent meal of the day should be the first one, whether you are working out or not during that day;

- Although this method doesn't normally lead to muscle loss (because it has just 16 hours of fasting period on a daily basis), you can also take BCAA (branch chain amino acids) just to prevent in possible muscle loss during a workout in the fasting period.

Once you decided that you want to try the Leangain method, there are some things you will need to set before going ahead with it:

1. You need to set when you start the fasting period, as you will need to have 16 hours without calorie intake. The best practice should be starting the fasting period in the evening. For instance, if you have the last meal of the day at 6 pm, you should be able to enter in the fasted state at 6 am. If you have the first meal of the day at 10 am, then the period between 6 am and 10 am should be the best time for training;

2. Once the fasting period is set, you will need to set the feeding time. You can set it by following the example above, from 10 am to 6 pm. Once you get used to fasting, you can extend the fasting period and decrease the feeding time, if you want more results. Therefore, you can have the fasting period around 18

hours, and the eating window for 6 hours;

3. Decide when it's the best time for training. You can adjust this method to your daily schedule, so if you work from 9 am to 6 pm, probably the best time to work out is in the morning, between 7 am and 8:15 - 8:30 am, assuming that you had your last meal at 7 pm the previous day.

The best way for the program to work is to not plan your feeding window when you normally sleep and also to take some BCAAs. Since most people are simply terrified about fasting for the long term, but a 16 hour fast is something very doable. All you need is self-discipline and to stay away from harmful food, like junk-food and other highly processed food with little to nothing nutrient value. Fasting for a long time is quite discouraging, and most people renounce it, but fasting for 16 hours can be something that anyone can do. Squeezing 3 meals into an 8-hour feeding window, may not be the best thing to do, as you don't want to exaggerate with the calories you consume, so you will need to figure it out which meal you will have to quit. Most of the nutritionists would agree that breakfast should be the meal you can skip, in order to make your fasting program work. Although plenty of people think that breakfast is the most important meal of the day, and it shouldn't be skipped, this is actually false. Having your first meal later during the day can have impressive positive effects on your body and health. Fasting in the morning determines your body to run on fat cells, so it starts to burn fats. However, the fat burning process is not the only benefit of Intermittent Fasting, as a detailed list of benefits can be seen in this subchapter.

The Warrior Diet is inspired by the lifestyle of the Spartan warriors from Ancient Greece. It was developed by Ori Hofmekler, a man who put his experience from the Israeli Military into practice. This fasting program splits the day into just 4 hours of eating period, correlated with a 20-hour fasting period. The reason why it's called the warrior diet is that in Ancient times, during wars, the warriors didn't have time for 3 meals during the regular day. Instead, they could only eat one massive meal and fight for the rest of the day. This was a really intense and difficult practice, but it had very good results for the warriors. Nowadays, you don't have to be at war to try this program, but you will need to narrow your feeding period to just 4-6 hours. You simply can't have two meals during this period, but you need to make sure that you consume the right type of food to cover your macronutrient necessary for the day and you have to do that with one meal. During the fasting period of 18-20 hours, you can only consume water and a minimum amount of snacks (just fruits or veggies, not chips or sweets), but you will also need to be very active, to burn calories, or in this case the fat tissue. The fasting period is long enough for the body to burn a higher amount of fat cells, so it can be very recommended for the fat burning process. Just like the Leangains method (16/8 fast), the warrior diet is a daily fasting process, but it's a bit more radical, as you can burn more fat using this procedure. The longer you fast, the more fat you burn. As long as there is fat to burn, the body will not try different energy sources during fasting, so you don't have to worry about muscle loss.

There are a few rules you will need to follow when trying this method:

- you will need to fast for at least 18 to 20 hours on a daily basis.

- if you enjoy having snacks, then you need to restrain yourself during the fasting period, as you can only consume moderate amounts of fruits or veggies.

- you will have to cover your protein intake with just one meal. This sounds like a very challenging task, especially because all bodies need a certain amount of proteins just to maintain the muscle mass. The general rule of thumb is 1 gram of protein reported to your body weight in pounds.

- getting all the calories you need in one meal can be a pretty challenging task, but this is what you will have to do during this program. So, make sure you have a consistent meal, in order to have the necessary calories.

Instructions

- establish when you want to have the eating period, whether you want it at breakfast, lunch or dinner;

- set how long you want the feeding window to last, 4 or 6 hours;

- decide if you want to consume snacks during the fasting period, as you can only have small portions of fruits or veggies, and possibly smoothies or protein shakes.

There are a few things you will have to avoid when trying this method. You can see them below:

- forget about sweets, pastries or chips, as the diet completely forbid them;

- avoid any meals during the fasting period. You can only have small snacks in terms of fruits, veggies, smoothies, or protein shakes;

- never change the time of the feeding period. If you have the eating window around dinner, don't change it to breakfast the next day, as it significantly decreases the fasting period.

You simply can't talk about Intermittent Fasting without the **Eat Stop Eat Diet**, developed by Brad Pilon. This program suggests a day of fast during a one-week period. The fasting period is now extended to 24 hours, but its frequency is now once per week. This is probably the easiest fasting program, as it can be tried by most of the healthy people or beginners. There is only one rule you will have to obey: don't eat anything for 24 hours, just drink water during this period. When it comes to the food you eat, there aren't any special requirements, however, avoiding junk-food and highly processed foods are very recommended. Fasting works better with physical exercise, and if you think that the body enters the fasted state 12 hours after the last meal, you will need to have an intense workout on the fasting day, as you can burn fats easier. If you are planning to try Intermittent Fasting, then most likely you would need to start with this program. It will give you a glimpse what IF is, and it would definitely convince to try it furthermore, or it will arouse the curiosity in you to try different other fasting methods.

The Alternate Day Fast is a very interesting program developed by Dr. James B. Johnson. This fasting program involved having a 12-hour feeding period, followed by a 36-hour fasting period. This program is designed to maximize the effects of Intermittent Fasting, as this is the program with the longest set fasting period. It is said that the longer you fast, the easier your body will burn fats. Since this is probably the only famous fasting program created by a nutritionist, it can be tried by a large variety of people. This program is not linked with training so you can try it without working out. As usual, the program works better if you also associate it with physical exercise. There are some simple rules you will need to follow:

1. You will have to respect the fasting period of 36 hours;

2. Eat as normal as possible during the eating window;

3. Although you can eat anything you want, you will need to avoid the excesses of highly processed food or any type of food considered caloric bomb.

When trying this Intermittent Fasting method, you will need to set up a few things:

- determine when you want to have the feeding period. It's highly recommended to have it as early in the morning as possible. If you consider having your first meal at 8 am, and your last meal at 8 pm, you will have the next meal at 8m the other day;

- After your last meal, the 36 hour-fast period takes place. If you have the feeding window on Monday from 8 am to 8 pm, that means that the fasting period will last from 8 pm on Monday until 8 am on Wednesday. Basically, you can eat for half of the day and fast for one day and a half. The fasting period can occur more than once during the week, so you can actually allow the body plenty of chances to burn fat.

Since a pure 36-hour fast is extremely difficult for the body (with having just water), this program allows you to consume some food during the fasting period. You can consume food of up to 20% of your normal calorie intake.

Intermittent Fasting is more about when you eat than what you eat. However, this doesn't mean that you can eat absolutely anything. In order to make this program work for you, you will have to be careful about what you eat. There are many nutritionists who recommend LCHF (low carbs high fats) diet. Still, not everyone knows how many carbs, fats, or proteins a food type contains. To make things easier for you, below there are a few food types that are highly recommended with Intermittent Fasting.

1. Avocado
2. Fish
3. Cruciferous Vegetables (broccoli, cauliflower, Brussels sprouts, etc.)
4. Potatoes
5. Legumes and Beans
6. Food Rich in Probiotics (kraut, kombucha, kefir and so on)
7. Berries
8. Eggs
9. Nuts
10. Whole Grains

These are the main food groups recommended being consumed in the Intermittent Fasting process. When it comes to the types of food which you will need to avoid as much as possible, it all comes down to logic and common sense. Any type of highly processed food should be avoided, junk-food especially and also snacks. Also, sweets or any other food type or drink very rich in salt and sugar should be avoided as much as possible. Sugar should be replaced with stevia, sweets with fruits or smoothies and for salt, sea salt is the most recommended type of salt in this case. Highly processed foods have little to no nutrient value, but very high calories. You have to consume higher quantities to cover the macronutrients your body requires, but you end up eating too many calories. This is why they have to be avoided as much as possible.

Usually, after 24 hours of fasting, your cells start to recycle more and more old components, but also to break down the wrong proteins associated with Alzheimer's or other illnesses. This process is called autophagy. "Autophagy is an important process for cellular and tissue rejuvenation – it removes damaged cellular components including misfolded proteins. Fasting activates the AMPK signaling pathway and inhibits mTOR activity, which in turn activate autophagy. This only begins to happen naturally, however, when you substantially deplete your glucose stores and your insulin levels begin to drop."[xxiv]

Let's just analyze some facts. Today, around 70% of the diseases known to humans are caused by the food we eat, correlated with a very passive lifestyle. Even the period when you eat the food can have harmful effects on your body, for instance, everyone should avoid eating just before sleeping. That's why something has to be done in order to become healthier and to prevent a wide variety of diseases. Intermittent Fasting can be the solution for this problem, and if you look at its benefits below, you can understand why:

a. Loss of body fat and weight through an enhanced fat burning process;

b. Decreased sugar levels and blood insulin;

c. There is the possibility to reverse type 2 diabetes;

d. Enhanced concentration and mental clarity;

e. Increased energy;

f. Enhanced growth hormone, at least in the short term;

g. Better cholesterol level;

h. Possible lower risk of Alzheimer's disease;

i. Potential anti-aging effect;

j. Cellular cleansing triggering through activation of autophagy;

k. Decreased inflammation levels.

Intermittent Fasting can be practiced for different reasons like disease prevention, fat burning, anti-aging, psychological effect, better mental performance, and enhanced physical condition. When it comes to disease prevention, IF is not useful just for type 2 diabetes or Alzheimer's disease, it can also prevent a wide range of heart, liver, kidney diseases, as well as other neurodegenerative diseases and even cancer. This procedure trains the body to burn fats, so the fat loss is perhaps the most visible effect. Also, Intermittent Fasting promotes a healthy lifestyle, which can lead to a longer life. It's very clear that this procedure kept humans more concentrated and vigilant in the prehistoric day, as they had to adapt quickly to the environment and focus on finding food. Fasting and physical exercise can turn fat into muscles, which can make humans stronger, more mobile and agile, so in better physical condition. Other benefits may include increased control over your appetite (and blood sugar, of course) and faster metabolism.

Part Three – Autophagy Without Fasting

As mentioned in the previous chapter, autophagy can be induced by Intermittent Fasting and a keto diet. These programs set the body to run on fats, whether it's the fat stored in your body and the fats you are consuming, or just the fat reserves. However, there are other ways to induce autophagy or factors that can influence it. Autophagy can also be induced by High-Intensity Interval Training (also known as HIIT), Protein Fast, but also sleep can favor this state.

HIIT

Autophagy is a domain that fascinates plenty of researchers and will probably fascinate for many years to come. That's why some scientists studied different ways to induce it. So far, we found out that Intermittent Fasting and Ketosis are doing a great job at inducing it. However, some researchers were convinced that physical exercise could also induce autophagy. Dr. Izumi Tabata, a Japanese researcher, conducted a study on 2 different groups to discover the differences between aerobic fitness and training intensities. This was in 1996, and all the participants used cycling ergometers for a 6 weeks training period. During this study, Dr. Izumi Tabata also measured the VO2 max levels, which represents the rate of oxygen consumption during physical training.

- There was a control group with just 60 minutes of moderate-intensity training 5 times per week at just 70% VO2 max. This is the low-intensity steady state cardio or LISS;

- The other group tried the HIIT approach (High-Intensity Interval

Training), having 20/10 sessions at 170% VO2 max, repeated 8 times. This means alternating the high-intensity exercise of very short rest breaks. A 20 seconds exercise followed by 10 seconds rest and repeated 8 times. The whole training lasted for 4 minutes.

After 6 weeks, the results were just incredible. The control group had 1800 minutes of training, compared to just 120 minutes of training for the HIIT group. The results showed that the VO2 max for the LISS group increased from 53 +/- 5 ml kg-1 min-1 to 58 +/-3 ml. kg-1. min 1, however, there wasn't much difference for their anaerobic capacity. The individuals in the HIIT group enhanced their VO2 max by 7 ml.kg-1, min-1, and their anaerobic fitness also increased by 28%.

This study also showed that HIIT is way more effective when it comes to causing physiological adaptations, and on top of that, it's way more time efficient than LISS. If you think about it, this makes perfect sense, as your body will have a much better response if you apply weight stress. You will have significantly more results if you lift something very heavy a few times than if you lift something very easy for too many times. There are also some other implications of the Tabata study that will need to be covered:

1) There was a significant improvement of the VO2 max levels for the LISS group. The body of those involved in this group got more efficient by working out at lower intensities, so they could easily get more intense training. Still, their bodies were becoming fitter as they were used to work at low intensities.

2) The subjects of the HIIT group managed to improve their VO2 max a bit more, they started at a lower level, but there is still room to improve this indicator. On the LISS group, the subjects were fitter, and it was already a lot more difficult to

notice any improvements.

3) The VO2 max level was still lower at the end of the study for the HIIT group compared to the LISS group. The HIIT group didn't become a lot fitter, but their relative fitness improved more.

However, the HIIT group had improved anaerobic and aerobic fitness, something that you can't say regarding the LISS group. Imagine if the HIIT group trained longer than 4 minutes, what impact that would have on their fitness. Unless you are looking to have much better endurance, there is no need to do hours of cardio at the gym. An average person trying to be fitter and healthier, the high-intensity interval training is a method way more efficient for exercise. It also saves you plenty of time, if you are stressed about time, but also determine a better metabolic and preserve your joints.

Tabata training and HIIT are just methods of endurance training. "Both of them are more intense, they burn muscle glycogen, improve insulin sensitivity, and stimulate the sympathetic nervous system. In fact, HIIT may lead to similar physiological adaptations in terms of muscle growth than resistance training. Not entirely, but it's not going to hinder the beneficial muscle building signals as much as cardio would."[xxv]

Mixing strength training with a lot of endurance training, may not be the best option, as your body will not find the time and resources to adapt to both pieces of training properly, so you will not achieve any of that. It's like trying to catch two rabbits at once, something that is not possible (at least to a man). In order to have better fitness condition in the long term, you will need to focus on HIIT and endurance training because you will have better results. If you think about the prehistoric humans (in hunting mode), they were stronger than us not because they walked all they (low-intensity training), but because they ran from large carnivore animals or towards their prey.

After fasting, physical exercise in the second factor in terms of effectiveness to enhance mitochondrial function and biogenesis through the same pathways of FOXO proteins and AMPK. HIIT raises the mitochondria's capability to produce energy by 69% at senior people and 49% in younger adults. Since HIIT and endurance training are amongst the most difficult methods of exercise, you can't train for around 75 minutes at the same intensity. Also, your workout shouldn't last just 4 minutes, like in the Tabata study. A 30-minutes workout per day should be more than enough to have serious autophagic effects. However, muscles are stimulated more during high-intensity workouts, so if you are worried about muscle loss, then you should know that the best way to prevent muscle waste or sarcopenia (loss of skeletal muscle) is to combine HIIT with endurance training. You will notice your muscles growing, and your fat tissue slowly decreasing. This is probably the best way to enhance your quality of life using physical exercise.

Protein Fast

Fasting seems to be more about scheduling your meals than about restraining yourself from consuming different types of food. Of course, it's highly recommended to associate fasting with a well-balanced diet, in which you have to cut down most of the carbs you consume. Most of the nutritionists would recommend the LCHF (low carbs high fats) diet, basically the keto diet. However, the keto diet only focuses on reducing carbs, as it is a way to induce autophagy. Well, glucose can also come from proteins, and consuming proteins can prevent the autophagy state. This is why some nutritionist recommended to also cut down on proteins, not just on carbs. In order to achieve this, they invented a special plan which involves lowering the daily protein consumption to 15 grams or even less. This program is called protein fast. It's known that the body needs to consume a certain amount of proteins to maintain its own muscle mass and lowering that consumption can lead to muscle loss. However, this can also be prevented. There are plenty of foods you can see in the supermarket that have labels with nutritional value on them. On that label, you should be able to see the protein level of the food. In the case of fruits or veggies, it is even harder to find out the protein level they have, as there is no label on it which can inform the consumer about that. You will need to inform yourself about all the food you are eating and its nutritional value because you can consume some food that you thought doesn't contain any proteins, but in fact, it does. That's why you need to be careful and get informed.

1) Search the internet for information, as even veggies can have protein levels. Of course, beans are known for their high proteins, but there are also other fruits and vegetables containing proteins, even broccoli has proteins;

2) Food regulations insist that labeled food needs to have nutritional value displayed. Usually, this information is displayed for a certain amount, e.g., proteins in 100 grams. You may be consuming more than 100 grams, so you need to do the right math, in order to find out exactly how much proteins you are having;

3) You can easily find out what food types have no proteins at all so you can exclude them from your diet. By doing this, you won't have to worry about the

protein limit of 15 grams per day. If you rule out proteins, make sure you don't replace them with carbs, as you need to keep the carbohydrate level to a minimum.

Fasting is known for having positive impacts on your body, like fat loss and detox. Protein fast has almost the same effects. You can practice it once a week, not every day, and allow your digestive system to run a self-maintenance process. If water fasting (when you only consume water) is recommended once a week, for your body to work even better, protein fasting has a similar effect and should be tried only once a week, as protein deprivation in a continuous form is not something recommendable. Decreasing protein consumption will generate autophagy (or self-digestion, how many refer to it) if performed once per week. So, you will be eating your own fat and proteins. "This is important not just for fat loss, but also for your cellular repair functions. Your enzymes from your pancreas and liver, in addition to breaking down and excreting toxins, have a secondary role of removing debris from the cells in your body."[xxvi]

But that's not all, as protein fasting can also have a positive effect on the mitochondrial function, leading to better sleep in time. A study conducted in 2013 by a team of scientists showed that autophagy is necessary for healthy brain cell mitochondria.[xxvii] Ketones are also important, as they act as fuel for mitochondria.

Autophagy is considered the body's natural self-cleaning process because it recycles the old and junk cells and turns them into energy. In time, there are oxidized parts, damaged proteins, and dead organelles accumulating in cells, which has a negative impact on the cell function and also favors aging. Autophagy makes the body perform better, and this leads indirectly to maintain the muscle mass in better shape than ever. There are a few main factors that trigger autophagy, but probably the most effective ones are fasting and lowering the protein intake. Limiting the protein intake once a week is even a better way to activate autophagy because it forces your cells to find all alternatives to recycles the proteins. As they ran an in-depth search (or scan), they can find toxins in the cell's cytoplasm. Protein fasting has similar benefits to Intermittent Fasting, as you can discover that protein deprivation can lower the mTOR and insulin level. "Remember, stomping down mTOR so its secretion can spring back up is key to building muscle."[xxviii] However, you will need to keep the protein deprivation on a short-term basis, as if practiced on a long-term basis, it can have harmful effects on your body and brains. That's why being vegan is not a very good option. Water fasting may be the easiest way to do this, but if you find it very harsh, you can also try the protein fast. It can have the same effects as water fasting, with less hunger. Limiting the protein intake in that day to just 15 grams may be a bit harsh, but it's totally doable, and the best part, it doesn't have any side effects, if applied on a healthy body.

Protein fasting may not be for everyone, depending on your health conditions you may need to ask a doctor first before attempting this diet. Most specialists would agree that this plan is not for pregnant women. However, extensive studies have not revealed if other categories of people should avoid protein fast. Most likely, the categories of people that can't practice Intermittent Fasting or a keto diet should also avoid the protein fast program. The shopping list should include approximately the same food types as the keto diet, but less extensive, as you are trying it for just one day per week.

Sleep can also influence the autophagy process, mostly because that's when this process happens. Getting the proper sleeping hours can help the autophagy process, but you don't want to sleep all the time, as you need to have an active lifestyle. A normal process should sleep between 7 and 8 hours per day, providing plenty of time for autophagy to happen. Keeping to the same sleeping schedule also helps the autophagy process, so going to sleep and waking up at approximately the same hour helps.

Part Four – What You Will Need To Eat In Order To Induce Autophagy

Inducing autophagy may not be an easy task to do, but there are several ways to generate it. Intermittent Fasting may be the most difficult method to apply in order to induce autophagy, but you don't have to stick to this method completely. You can try a combination of Intermittent and Protein Fasting or the Alternate Day Fast (but without consuming any calories during the fasting period). It is known that autophagy usually happens within 24-36 hours after your last meal. Daily fasting really can't apply in this case, so you need something which lasts longer.

Plan A would mean the combination of Intermittent and Protein Fasting. It can great effects on your health and also on your fat tissue and will definitely induce autophagy. You can eat what you normally eat and compile special shopping for the Protein Fast day. Eating healthier is something that you would definitely want to do. Therefore, you will need to buy food types that have fewer carbs. Remember. the main goal of doing this is to train your body to run on fats. Therefore, try to avoid food types rich and carbs, especially sugar and starch, so you may need to rule out bread, pastries, pasta, potatoes, or rice. You can replace potatoes and rice, with different veggies which are low in carbs, or brown rice. Something that you will need to avoid during a diet is to compensate the caloric deprivation of the fasting period. That's why you will eat as normal as possible and try to avoid excess calories, even though you will be doing fasting.

The following plan doesn't include a detailed menu, but it does have the kind of ingredients you will need to consume. The main principle of the food you will be waiting is Low Carb

High Fats. You can also be a bit careful with the protein intake, but the food you will eat will have to be rich in fats.

Monday

Start your day with a consistent breakfast. An omelet with herbs seems to be the right choice. You can avoid eating meat at this meal, especially if it's processed, so sausages are definitely out of the question. The protein and fat intake are covered by this meal, so you don't need any addition at all, perhaps just some high-fat cheese. As a drink of choice, you can have coffee or tea but without sugar. You can have instead cream in your coffee, and when it comes to tea, you need to consume green, black, or herbal tea. Try to avoid fruity teas, as they are too sweet for what you plan to accomplish.

At lunch, you can fry some veggies in butter, along with some chicken breast. For veggies, you would need to have broccoli, carrots, peas, cauliflower, asparagus, etc. You can have these fresh or frozen, and slowly fry them in butter. When adding spices, make sure you keep the salt level as low as possible. As for meat, 150-200 grams of a chicken breast should be more than enough.

For dinner, you will need to try high-fat yogurts and nuts. Cashews may not be the right option, as they have a higher carb level, but walnuts may be the right option in this case. The caloric intake during the day is not very high, but in order to burn more fat, you will need to exercise also. The best time for your workout is during the morning on an empty stomach. The most important factors that help to induce autophagy are fasting, protein limitation, exercise, and sleep. To recap, on Monday morning you wake up after a restful sleep (7-8 hours), and you start exercising or go to the gym on an empty stomach (after a cup of coffee). You can burn fats easier that way. After training, you will have the first meal of the day, the consistent omelet with herbs and possibly high-fat cheese. Then you just have the other meals with approximately 4 hours gap between them. Therefore, a regular day would look like:

6:30 am - wake up, then drink coffee;

7 to 7:30 am - exercise. During this period is highly recommended to try HIIT;

8 to 8:30 am - breakfast;

12:30 to 1:30 pm - lunch;

3:30 - snack time. Please use fruits for in this case. Avocados, kiwis, apples, pineapples, oranges, and other fruits are highly indicated. Try to avoid really sweet fruits like berries; they should only be used on top of the cream. Nuts are highly recommended, with the exception of cashews because they have a higher carb value.

5:30 to 6 pm - dinner;

9 pm - evening exercise;

10:30 to 11 pm - bedtime.

Tuesday

Start your day with a bowl of nutritious breakfast cereals, out of whole grains. You can use semi-skimmed or whole milk, but don't exaggerate, as milk is known to be a source of carbs;

At lunch, you can have some baby potatoes with grilled pork sirloin, and cabbage salad on the side. The pork sirloin can have a maximum of 150 grams, as it has a bit of fat, but it doesn't have to be too proteic. Baby potatoes are not that rich in carbs, as other types of potatoes are, but still, you can only consume a few of them. The cabbage salad makes a nice addition to the meal, even if you don't use olive oil on it (which is the most recommended oil when it comes to fats).

For dinner, you can serve a Greek salad, on

which you will have to make sure you put plenty of olive oil. Instead of feta cheese, you can use a fatter cheese, but make sure it's natural, not highly processed.

You can stick to the same schedule as for the previous day, waking up, working out, and having the meals at approximately the same hours.

Wednesday

This day you can have two slices of toast with high-fat butter spread. You can serve next to a cup of herbal tea but without any sugar.

For lunch, you can have brown rice with mushrooms, to avoid meat, and to keep the carbs intake as low as possible. Brown rice is known to have fewer calories than normal rice.

At dinner, you can have soup, in which carrots, celery, broccoli, brown rice, and other veggies can be used as ingredients. Keeping to the schedule, sleeping well, and also working out is essential in order to induce autophagy. Eating the right fruits as snacks are also very important; berries and bananas are not that recommended in this case.

Thursday

Start your day with high-fat yogurt and muesli. It should provide the fat intake you need for the day and should be between the carbs and protein limits.

For lunch, you can serve Asian Noodles with sesame dressing, a very interesting meal that should prepare you for the next day. You can use kelp noodles, a type of pasta which is lower in carbs, and besides that, you should be able to see carrots, bell pepper, garlic, and possibly other veggies. Just before dinner, you can change the fruits snacks with smoothies.

At dinner, you can have baked baby potatoes with chives and butter, keeping the carb intake at a decent level and making sure the fats level is high enough.

You can skip the gym during this day, but you can still exercise a bit in the evening. Besides this, you can stick to the standard schedule.

Friday

In some religions, Friday is a designated day for fasting before major holidays. You can use Friday as your fasting day for the week. The first time you try the program, you should make Friday the Protein Fast day. In order to consume less than 15 grams of protein for this day, you will need to have a special menu for the day. Although you are limiting your protein consumption, don't let this stop you from training. In order for autophagy to be more effective, you will need to work out during this day, so you have to get back to the normal daily schedule.

You will need to skip breakfast, but you can drink coffee or tea (green tea, preferably). There shouldn't be any trace of proteins in this drink, so no cream, milk, butter at all. It goes without saying that sugar is forbidden.

At lunch, which by the way, has to be after 15-18 hours after your last dinner, you can try baked carrot fries with iceberg salad. You can have dinner 5 to 6 hours after your lunch. At dinner, you can have guacamole with baked sweet potatoes.

The following week, you can swap the protein fast day with a "pure" water fasting day, in order to have better results on your fat burning process.

Saturday

After a day of fasting, you need proteins again, so the meat is back on the menu. However, you will not need to exaggerate with it, so it's better to have just at lunch.

An herb omelet with high-fat cheese should get you started for the day.

At lunch, you can have a mix of veggies with a beef steak. Beef should not be more than 150-

200 grams.

For dinner, you can have a celery soup. Since you are increasing your caloric intake, you will need to stick to the normal schedule and make sure you work out as well.

Sunday

You should start the day with 2 slices of bread and high-fat butter spread on them and also enjoy some herbal or green tea, without any sugar of course.

For lunch, you can have brown rice with grilled pork sirloin. The piece shouldn't be more than 150-200 grams, and you can also have a cabbage salad on the side.

At dinner, you can enjoy high-fat yogurt with walnuts.

Well, this is plan A, which can be easier to apply. However, plan B involves the alternate day fast, so you should have two fasting periods per week. This plan limits your feeding window at just 12 hours, and it's followed by 36 hours of fasting. During the 12 hours feeding window, you can follow an LCHF diet, with 3 meals per day, and the fasting period should only consist of drinking water. This method is a lot harder than plan A, but it will definitely induce autophagy, as you are fasting for more than 24 hours and you consume fewer carbs and proteins. Please remember to sleep 7-8 hours per day and even though is very hard, try very intensive training methods like HIIT.

The Alternate Day Fast is a program developed by Dr. James B. Johnson, and in normal circumstances is a softer fasting program, because it allows some snacks during the fasting period, but the version you need to try it's a bit different than the original one. Also, the original program allows you to eat anything you want, making the program very accessible for a wide variety of people. To adapt the alternate fasting day program to induce autophagy, you may need to change what you are eating during the feeding period and make sure that you consume only water during the 36 hours fasting period. For this diet, you will need to:

a. Establish your feeding period to 12 hours. This is something very doable, as during this feeding period you can have 3 meals. Let's say you have your first meal at 8 am and the last one at 8 pm. The normal Alternate Day Fast Program includes normal meals, but in order to induce autophagy, you may need to have an LCHF diet, so levels of carbs and even proteins;

b. If you had the last meal at 8 pm on Monday, you would have the next meal on Wednesday at 8 am. This means a 36 hour "pure" fast, in which you can only consume water. It may be a very difficult period, but it's still doable. People can last on water fasting for tens or hundreds of days, without having health side effects. If the original program suggests, you have to have during fasting periods 20% of the calories you normally consume during the feeding period. However, we suggest a more radical approach with 0 calories in the fasting period, although it lasts for 36 hours. This will give the body plenty of time to induce autophagy and recycle the damaged parts of cells.

Autophagy is a beneficial process, so why not induce it twice a week. You can see below how Plan B looks like, so prepare yourself because it's quite radical.

Monday

Breakfast at 8 am, you can start your day with an herb omelet with extra cheese. At lunch, you can have roasted baby potatoes with grilled pork sirloin and a salad on the side. At dinner, you can have high-fat yogurt with walnuts. You can also have two snacks during the day, between breakfast and lunch, and between lunch and dinner. Snacks can only consist of fruits or veggies so you will need to try avocado, pineapple, kiwi, watermelon, apples, mango, or other fruits. By 8 pm you finished eating your dinner so you can prepare yourself to fast.

Monday 8 pm to Wednesday at 8 am - fasting period. Make sure you consume just water.

Wednesday 8 am - breakfast. You can try 2 slices of toast with butter spread, with green or herbal tea (no sugar, of course). Meat should be present in every day you eat, so for lunch, you can have fried vegetables with grilled chicken breast. You can use butter to fry the veggies. For dinner, you can try a light soup, like the BBB soup (brown rice, broccoli, and bok choy).

Wednesday 8 pm to Friday at 8 am - fasting. Stick to the same rules as the previous fast.

Friday 8 am - breakfast. You can try a bowl of

cereals, but make sure they are whole grains. You can use a moderate quantity of semi-skimmed or whole milk, but try to keep it minimal, as milk has carbs. For lunch, you can try roasted baby potatoes with beef steak and cabbage salad on a side. At dinner, you can have a Greek salad with high-fat cheese instead of feta.

For the weekend, you can follow the normal feeding rules. You can also have some fish instead of beef (salmon or tuna is great in this case). You can even have cream soups, Asian Noodles, and other salads. Occasionally, you can switch from fruits (snacks) to smoothies or protein shakes. Plan B shouldn't be tried on a regular basis, as it's very drastic. It should probably be tried twice or three times per year.

Types of Food Which Can Induce Autophagy

People trying to achieve autophagy perhaps are wondering what food they will need to eat in order to induce autophagy. Without any doubt, the type of food you eat can favor or suppress autophagy. The more natural the food is, the more likely is to induce autophagy. However, when it comes to this process, it's more about the nutrient density the food has than the caloric density. That's why low carbs and high-fat diets are known to induce autophagy. Also, lowering the protein intake should also get you there. It's highly important to know exactly what you can eat or drink, in order for this process to be activated. Green tea, coffee, pepper, and ginger are known as the most beneficial food types and drinks when it comes to the autophagy process. So, in order for your body to recycle the damaged cell parts and organelles, you will have to consume certain foods and drinks.

Let's start with green tea, which is considered by a few people the healthiest drink after mineral water. The main polyphenol in green tea is the Epigallocatechin gallate (shortly known as EGCG), which is known to have plenty of health benefits. "Too much green tea, however, may cause anxiety and heart palpitations because of the high caffeine content, which makes using green tea extracts or EGCG supplements a more convenient way to add extra polyphenols to your diet. Doses above 500 mg may become problematic."[xxix] The EGCG from green teas is known to suppress the IGF-1 (Insulin growth factor 1) stimulated lung cancer. Other herbal teas are also known as low autophagic foods, but just green tea has the EGCG polyphenol which can stimulate hepatic autophagy. However, that's not all, as the green tea has a special substance that can easily melt fat from your body. This special substance is the L-Theanine, which is an amino acid known for its alertness boosting effect, although it's not as powerful as in coffee. The caffeine release from the L-Theanine is more long-lasting and subtle, and this makes the green tea an interesting addition to your morning coffee.

Another low autophagy food or drink is coffee. "Coffee induces autophagy and has benefits on cellular metabolism. It can also stabilize blood sugar, enhance fat oxidation, and protect against neurodegeneration, which makes it the perfect drink for fasting. However, too much caffeine will raise cortisol, which can promote inflammation and visceral fat formation around your belly."[xxx] Also, in the modern-day standard diet, coffee is the primary source of polyphenols. When fasting, hot coffee can make you absorb fewer nutrients because of tannins and caffeine. Through the autophagy-lysosomal pathway, coffee can stimulate lipid metabolism. The excess of caffeine consumption may lead not only to increased cortisol but also to higher levels of insulin and blood glucose. This is the reason why abusing coffee may interfere with your fast. The recommended coffee consumption should be around 2-4 cups per day.

Another low autophagy food is the black pepper, as it has piperine, a compound capable of inducing autophagy. However, not only ingredients can stimulate autophagy, as also the cayenne pepper is known as a low autophagic food because of its capsaicin, a compound who favors the activation of autophagy.

The food types or drinks capable of inducing autophagy are:

- berries and fruits (raspberries, blueberries, strawberries, blackberries, elderberries, cranberries, and cherries);

- herbs and spices (rosemary, basil, coriander, cilantro, thyme, cardamom, turmeric, cinnamon, ginger, ginseng, black pepper, cayenne pepper);

- drinks and beverages (coffee, all teas, especially black or green, red wine, white wine, gin, vermouth, vodka).

Supplements Which Can Help You With Autophagy

The food types should do their magic and should be able to induce autophagy; however, if you are interested in better results when it comes to autophagy, you can use other supplements as well. Some of the most effective supplements, in this case, are the nicotinamide and the resveratrol.

Also known as niacin, nicotinamide is an alternative form of vitamin B3, which can be converted into nicotinamide adenine dinucleotide (NAD+), a helper molecule or a coenzyme. Some of the functions of NAD+ are:

- converts food into energy;

- repairs damaged DNA;

- strengthens the cells' defense systems;

- setting the circadian rhythm and internal clock of the body.

As you are getting older, the NAD+ level also decreases, that's why you may need to get supplements containing this form of vitamin B3. If you are wondering why you need more of it, it has been showed that an increased level of NAD+ could slow down the aging process and also can significantly decrease the risk of many chronic diseases. In more details, this coenzyme can protect brain cells (so, therefore, it can be useful to prevent Parkinson's and Alzheimer's disease), may be very useful for a healthy aging process, can lower the risk of heart diseases, cancer and it can also help with weight loss. The daily requirement is around 250-300 mg per day.

Resveratrol is a plant compound which can be used for inducing autophagy. It's from the stilbenoid class, and it's a type of phytoalexin and a natural phenol, produced by a few plants in response to injury. This substance can be found in food types like red grapes, dark chocolate, peanut butter, and blueberries. Also, it can be found in red wines. The daily recommended dosage is 250 mg.

Other supplements highly recommended for autophagy are the Omega 3s, Vitamin D-3, and Magnesium.

"Omega 3s - The more omega-6 fatty acids you consume, the more omega 3s you may need. A healthy dose of omega-3s is 1000-3000 mg/day. Research shows that more than 5000 mg doesn't seem to have any added benefits. For EPA and DHA, you should aim for a minimum of 250 mg and a maximum of 3000 mg/day in a combined dose. Eat wild fatty fish a few times a week."[xxxi] You can find omega-3s in fish oil, krill oil, cod liver oil, hempseed oil, wheat germ, and algae omega.

Vitamin D-3 is responsible for most of the functions in our body from metabolism to DNA repair. It can prevent infective, autoimmune, and cardiovascular diseases. Vitamin D should normally be obtained directly from the sun. However, in some regions of the globe, it's not quite possible in some seasons. The minimum requirement for an adult should be around 2000 IUs of vitamin D, whilst the maximum supported level should be between 4000-5000 IU/day. Extremely high levels of vitamin D, between 10000-40000 IUs is very toxic. Vitamin D supplements can come in the form of oil or capsules.

"Magnesium - It comprises 99% of the body's mineral content and governs almost all physiological processes. Magnesium helps to build bones, enables nerves to function, and is essential for the production of energy from food. Deficiencies can drive cardiovascular disease, depression, and headaches."[xxxii] The recommended daily dosage is 400 mg, and this is quite important if you live an active lifestyle, as you may experience muscle cramps or other problems related to muscles.

However, there are several other minerals and nutrients that you need to cover when being in the autophagy state. Some minerals and micronutrients zinc, potassium, vitamin K, and all the B vitamins are vital for your energy and health. You can see them below:

- Calcium has the RDA of 1000-1200 mg and is extremely important for your bones, as it's responsible for strengthening them;

- Choline with 425-550 mg RDA is useful for your attention and cognitive function. Also, it has a positive impact on cholesterol transportation, methyl metabolism, and cell membrane;

- Iron is very important for hemoglobin transportation (helps with the oxygen transfer to cells and muscles). The RDA is 8-18 mg, a dosage which can be achieved just from food or supplements;

- Iodine is important for metabolism and thyroid functioning. The RDA is 150 mcg, and most people are deficient when it comes to this mineral;

- Potassium has the minimum requirement at 2000 mg per day, and the RDA is 4700 mg/day but is easy to be found in leafy vegetables and avocados.

- Selenium is crucial for energy and hormones production, especially testosterone. The RDA is around 55 mcg, but the optimal level should be between 100 and 300 mcg;

- Zinc is important for cell growth, defending the immune system and protein synthesis. The RDA is 8-12 mg/day.

Some of the main vitamins you will need to cover, in order to improve the functionality of your body are vitamin A, the B vitamin group (B1, B2, B3, B5, B6, B7, B9, and B12), vitamin C, vitamin E, and vitamin K.

Part Five – Changing Your Lifestyle

Autophagy is a process which can be induced by different factors. This chapter will not cover the pathways of autophagy AMPK and mTOR, but it will cover instead how to induce it, how to plan it in real life. As previously mentioned in this book, autophagy can be favored by Intermittent Fasting, Ketosis, HIIT, Protein Fasting, and Sleep.

How To Make Fasting A Way of Life?

Becoming healthier and more fit should be a primary goal that anyone should follow. Autophagy can help you achieve this goal, as it's responsible for destroying and recycling old and damaged cells parts, in order for your body to work better. It is usually linked with the fat burning process, as autophagy happens when the body runs on fat. It basically actions on the fat cells, in order to get the energy required for your brain and body. Ketosis and fasting can be intertwined, as ketosis is regarded as the first phase of Intermittent Fasting, during which ketones levels are higher. Ketosis is not the same thing as the keto-adaption process. The first term describes a metabolic state with appropriate levels of ketones and blood sugar. During this phase, the insulin level and blood sugar decreases, whilst the ketones levels are increasing. This is generated by the glucose deprivation, meaning that it took quite a while since the body last had its glucose required for energy. This substance can be found in all the carbs (and proteins as well) and is the primary source of energy for the body under "normal circumstances." Speaking of glucose intake, the modern-day diet relies heavily on carbs because we mainly consume processed food.

This means that the body mainly uses the glucose from the carbs, but the big problem is that it simply can't burn all the glycogen it gets, mainly because of the high carb intake, but also because of the passive lifestyle. Nowadays, around 70% of the diseases known to humans are caused by the food we eat, and high amounts of carbs can be blamed for this situation. In urban communities, where most people live, is kind of difficult to find natural and organic food, as everywhere you are bombarded by processed food. The sad truth is that most of the food we eat today is processed, and this comes with very high levels of carbs. What's even worse, is that these types of food have little to nothing nutritional value and causes addiction. In order to cover your daily nutritional needs, you have to eat more, but this means a caloric boom. Processed food is more caloric dense than nutrient dense, and this is a major disadvantage. When people are facing increased risks of chronical diseases like type 2 diabetes, heart, stomach, liver and kidney diseases, it's clear that something has to be done to change the way we eat and also what we eat. Studies indicate that in order to become healthier and also thinner, you would need to decrease the glucose level when eating. This can happen by cutting down on carbs and, in some cases, also means protein limiting. When not burned, glucose gets stored into your blood, increasing the insulin and blood sugar level. Carbs consumption is like a vicious circle, as you easily get hungry after consuming food rich in carbs, and you are craving for more. But these meals come with strings attached, as you will get higher glucose levels and eventually higher blood sugar and insulin level. In order to make a radical change, you will need to make your body burn fat, not glucose. As you probably already have blood sugar, you will need to stop eating so many carbs, and therefore, you will have less glucose to worry about. You can achieve this through fasting (restraining yourself from food) or through a special diet.

Traditional fasting means not consuming any food at all; some would not consume anything at all, just like religious fanatics during a special period, the Ramadan in the Islamic religion can be a perfect example. By not consuming anything at all, you are allowing your body to use the available glucose to be burnt, and once it has burned it all, the body will have to switch the energy source from glucose to fat. As the glucose level is decreasing, the same happens with the insulin level, setting it free to do its job and regulate the blood sugar. The body easily adapts to such changes, and since its glucose reserves are running out, it has to figure out a way to use a different fuel type. That's where ketones step in, which is the necessary tool to break down fat cells and release the energy from them. You need to easily make the difference between ketosis and the keto-adapted process, as ketosis represent the metabolic state during which the ketone bodies are multiplying. The keto-adapted process is responsible for switching the energy source from glucose to fat. You can be in a ketosis state, but still not running on fats and ketones for fuel.

Intermittent Fasting is more of a self-discipline process because it's about planning when to eat than what to eat. Limiting the feeding window to a limited amount of hours can give time for the body to process the food and use it for energy. However, when the body has already processed the food it has consumed, and it's not receiving anything else, it will start to look for a different alternative as fuel. The fat tissue is the most "to hand" option, and ketones can help extract the energy from it. If daily fasting has feeding and a fasting window, these terms are not the same with the fed and fasted state. The fed state represents the period of time required by your body to process the food it consumed, whilst the fasted state refers to the period after the fed state, during which the body doesn't have to process any food, and it's also not receiving any nutrients at all. The fasted state starts approximately 12 hours after the last meal, and, coincidence or not, that's when ketosis starts. In the fasted state, the ketones levels are increasing rapidly, whilst the blood sugar and insulin levels are decreasing. At this point, the body doesn't have available glucose to burn, and it's looking for alternative fuel. Also, this is the right moment to apply stress to your body, and by stress, you need to understand the physical exercise. This will force the fat burning process, will increase even more the ketones levels, and the insulin will take care of the stored glucose from your blood. This is how the keto-adaptation gets started when your body starts to run on fats. Since ketosis is considered the first phase of Intermittent Fasting, these 2 processes go "hand-in-hand," but ketosis can be achieved in a different way also, through a keto diet. Sticking to the IF process, if you want to achieve autophagy, you may need to fast for a longer period of time, as daily fasting may not be enough for autophagy. Fasting between 24 and 48 hours should normally induce autophagy, but this is not an exact science, as the fasting period required to trigger the autophagy period may be different from a person to another. Some people have tried fasting for a longer period, consuming just water. However, this method should only be tried as a last case scenario, as it can be pretty drastic to try it for a longer period of time. Most of the Intermittent Fasting benefits can be achieved after up to 72 hours of fasting, so there shouldn't be any reasons to fast longer than that. Autophagy will be triggered during this kind of fast, so you will get rid of the damaged proteins, organelles, and cell parts from your body and replace them with brand new ones. If you are worried about muscle loss, I have news for you. The growth hormone reaches incredible levels after 72 hours of fasting, so you will not only burn fat, but you will maintain your muscle mass. Getting more muscle mass depends on the protein intake and the intensity of training. 72 hours fast will not get you the performance you are looking for so you will not gain more muscles. You are not getting any proteins also, as you are consuming just water.

During the fasting process, you will have to train your brain to forget about food and to deal better with the hunger situations, as you will be experiencing starvation. There are softer fasting programs, which can also induce autophagy, so you will not have to rush into the hardest one. You can try several of them, depending on the difficulty level of the program. Some fasting methods would include the Leangains method (16 hours of fasting correlated with 8-hour feeding window), The Warrior Diet (4-6 hours of eating time, the rest is just pure fasting), Eat Stop Eat (or the 24 hours fast) and the Alternate Day Diet (12 hours feeding window/36 hours fasting period). The "purest" method of fasting is considered water fasting, but this is usually a long term fast and very radical, as you can't consume any calories at all. Officially, the feeding window of any fasting program doesn't have any special food requirements. Practically, in order for the program to be more effective, you will need to cut down on carbs, so you simply can't eat anything you want. Food types like bread, pasta, pastries, potatoes, or rice should be eliminated from your diet, or consumed in moderate amounts. You can try the daily fasting, or you can try fasting every other day or just once per week. Depending on your objective, you can select one of the available fasting programs. This procedure is not for everyone, so if you have a medical condition, perhaps Intermittent Fasting is not for you.

Another way to enter the ketosis phase is the keto diet; a special LCHF method focused on making your body run on fats. This type of diet replaces carbs with fats, so it lowers them to a minimum level, or perhaps just eliminates them completely. Intermittent Fasting mostly relies on starvation to induce autophagy. The keto diet relies on carbs deprivation to induce it. When it comes to carbs, you need to know that they are present in too many types of food, especially if it's processed. Carbs are divided into sugars in starch. Sugar is probably the most harmful ingredient on the face of the Earth. It's consumed on a global scale, and it has too many people addicted to it. The effects of sugar consumption are obvious for most people. Different governmental measures were taken in order to better inform the consumer of the risk of sugar, products are properly labeled so you can see the sugar level on it, and some governments have even applied an extra tax on products containing sugar. All of these measures were designated to lower the consumption of such products. Any processed product has a smaller or higher value of sugar, but there are a few which can be considered sugar bombs. You need to avoid consumption of soft drinks, fruit juices, sweets, candies, and so on. The other major carb type is represented by starch, which can be found in bread, pasta, pastries, rice, and potatoes. Moderate consumption, or even completely eliminating these types of food from the menu is desirable, although these types of food are amongst the most common and popular worldwide.

The keto diet significantly lowers the carb intake because they are the main source of glucose. However, glucose can be found in proteins as well, so lowering the protein level is also something that you need to do. The keto diet should have a ratio of just 5% carbs, 15% - 25% proteins, and the rest should consist of fats. This is the standard keto diet. There is also a version which involves a higher protein intake, but not higher than 35%, but also keeping the carbs level extremely low. The keto diet is capable of inducing autophagy, although through it the body gets fed. Autophagy is induced when the body runs on fat, and this is where the keto diet steps in. If Intermittent Fasting trains the body to consume the fat reserves, the keto diet trains the body to use the fat consumed through this diet, and once that's finished, to continue consuming fats from the fat reserves.

As mentioned above, the keto diet focuses more on food types with higher levels of fat. That's why you will need to include in your menu food types like avocado, olive oil, fish (especially salmon), meat (pork, beef or chicken), eggs, high-fat dairy products, fruits, leafy green veggies, legumes, nuts, berries and so on. Avocado should be present in any keto diet, as it has plenty of benefits for the fat burning process and for autophagy itself. When it comes to fish, make sure you consume the fatty kind of meat, salmon is perhaps the best example. Tuna is also a good alternative. When it comes to meat, you can go for the fattier ones, but still, you will need to consume them moderately, as there are also sources of proteins and glucose. The same rule applies for fish as well. Eggs are highly recommended during a keto diet so you can consume as many as you like, but still, don't exaggerate with them. High-fat dairy products should not be missing from any keto diet. You can consume in this case butter, yogurt, cream, or cheese, all high fat. Milk is not quite recommended, as it's also a source of carbs, regardless if it is semi-skimmed or whole milk. When it comes to fruits, you can include most of the fruits known to man, especially oranges, limes, lemons, apples, pineapples, mango, kiwi and all sorts of berries, as they are known for inducing autophagy. In terms of vegetables, the general rule is what grows over the ground. So, you can use plenty of lettuce, green salad, spinach, cauliflower, broccoli, Brussels sprouts, but also celery, carrots, onions, garlic, peppers, asparagus and many more. Nuts are very good for a ketogenic diet, so you can consume all kind of nuts in this diet, but also moderately.

Autophagy Without Fasting

If you are looking for a softer method to induce autophagy, then protein fasting is the method for you. Protein fasting is very similar to the keto diet as it has approximately the same food types allowed, but through this method, you are trying to use fewer proteins also, not just carbs. Glucose can be found in proteins also, so why take any chances and reduce the protein intake as well. This is not something recommended in the long run, but on the short term, it can have amazing results in terms of inducing autophagy (along with all the benefits that can come from inducing it). If a keto diet usually keeps the protein percentage around 15% - 25%, this method is bound to limit the protein consumption to just 15 grams per day. This means that you will mostly eat fats during the protein fast day, as carbs should also be consumed in very low amounts. This procedure should be tried once per week or even once per month. Protein deprivation has bad effects on the long run, but as it turns out, on a short-term basis, it can be a very useful tool for triggering autophagy. Since you are feeding the body a very small amount of proteins, this will allow the autophagy process to recycle any damaged protein, old cellular part, and organelles. Some specialists would consider that this process is even more effective at inducing autophagy than fasting itself. Since the protein fast seems to be diet derived from the keto diet, it's recommended to use a keto diet the rest of the days, to have better effects. This way, the protein fast should be a walk in the park, if you are already following a keto diet. The protein deprivation process should not be very difficult in this case, as the shopping list should not be affected too much by this fasting day. The protein fasting day involves skipping breakfast (drinking just coffee or tea, without any sugar or any proteins at all, so no milk or cream in the coffee or tea). For lunch, you can have a few veggies like lettuce with baked carrots, and for dinner, you can try some baked potatoes with guacamole. Very important, the lunch should be after 15 to 18 hours after your last meal and dinner should be after 5 to 6 hours after lunch.

Another method to induce autophagy is the high-intensity interval training, also known as HIIT. When it comes to burning fat, there is nothing compared to such high intensity or endurance training. This method involves having exercises of 20 seconds, followed by a 10 seconds break, then repeating the exercise 8 times. HIIT is probably the best option to increase the oxidative stress, as you will train your body to lift heavier stuff, in short term rounds, which have to be repeated several times, having just very limited and short breaks. This type of exercise will not let your body rest, as it will push itself to become better at endurance and at overall fitness. HIIT is even better than cardio, as it is more diversified, you can apply it to more muscle groups, whilst cardio can't be applied to many muscle groups. One major advantage of HIIT is the time-efficiency, as you will be able to work for more muscle groups in record time, assuming that you can keep the pace. If a normal workout at the gym is between 75 and 90 minutes, a very HIIT session should not last more than 30 minutes. Imagine having this session daily and how much fat you will burn. Exercise or physical stress is yet another factor that can induce autophagy. This is what HIIT does, as it boosts the fat burning process with incredibly intense exercises.

Sleep shouldn't be underestimated, as a proper restful sleep can be very important for the autophagy process. This is when this process happens, so you definitely want to give plenty of time for autophagy "to work its magic." You shouldn't exaggerate with sleeping, but you still need to find the right balance between sleep time and being awake time. The normal period of sleep for an adult is 7-8 hours, and this period should be respected, as you also need to have an active lifestyle, have great energy levels and to feel rested during the day. In order to avoid fatigue, you need to set your own sleeping schedule, and you need to stick to it. You should sleep for approximately 7-8 hours, wake up and go to sleep at approximately the same time. For example, you can go to sleep between 10:30 and 11:30 pm and wake up between 6:30 and 7:30 am. It makes sense that for a good night sleep, you will need to avoid late snacking.

In order to maximize the results of the autophagy process, you will need to combine all of the factors into one plan. You have Intermittent Fasting, Ketosis, Protein Fast, HIIT, and sleep. A good alternative would be having a daily fast and using a keto diet (a bit higher in proteins) for the feeding period. You can try the Leangains method of fasting, with 16 hours of fasting and 8 hours of feeding. A plan, in this case, would look something like this:

Normal fasting day:

7:30 am - wake up and drink coffee;

8 am to 8:30 am - HIIT training at the gym;

10 am - breakfast, use a keto recipe to prepare an LCHF breakfast. If you are preparing an herb omelet, you can add in some bacon, for extra fat and proteins;

noontime for a snack. You will have to eat some fruits or veggies and this case. Avocado, berries, apple, pineapple, mango, orange may be the right choice;

1:30 to 2 pm - lunch time. Meat should be on the menu, so make sure you have it in there. Grilled chicken breast and veggies fried (in butter) may be the right choice;

4 pm - the second snack of the day. You can try fruits or smoothies.

6 pm - dinner. You can try something like a Greek salad or soup.

9 pm - evening exercise

11 to 11:30 pm - going to bed

11:30 pm to 7:30 am the next day - sleeping

This plan can be respected in most days of the week, but you can have also a protein fast day on Friday. On such a day, you will stick to this plan, only change the diet of the day. You will need to skip breakfast and only stick to coffee in the morning but make sure you don't add any protein to it, so no cream, butter or milk. If the previous day you had dinner at 6 pm, you can have lunch at noon and dinner at 6 pm. For lunch, you can try a sweet potato-ginger soup, and for dinner, you can have buttered white rice with iceberg salad. During the weekend, you can get back at the normal schedule, with the 16/8 fasting (Leangains method), combined with a higher protein keto diet and of course, HIIT training. Combining all of these methods will enhance the autophagy activity leading to a better fat burning process, increased energy levels, lower insulin and blood sugar levels, better control over your appetite, an enhanced cognitive function (thus preventing neurodegenerative diseases like Alzheimer's and Parkinson's disease). Also, this method should prevent type 2 diabetes and lower the risk of heart, kidney, and liver diseases. As the plan indicates, you will need to consume coffee on a daily basis, you can also try green tea, but you will also need to consume berries or nuts during snacks, or black pepper as a condiment and also cayenne peppers. All these types of food and drinks are autophagic, and although the consumption of alcohol is not quite recommended, a glass of red wine during the weekend should have positive effects over the whole autophagy process.

Below you can see a more detailed list of food types and drinks capable of inducing autophagy:

- berries and fruits. In this category you would need to include all kind of berries like strawberries, blueberries, raspberries, blackberries, but also cherries;

- herbs and spices. You should eat black pepper, cayenne pepper, ginger, cinnamon ginseng, cilantro, thyme, basil, and rosemary;

- drinks and beverages. In this category, you can find coffee, herbal and green tea, red wine, vermouth, gin, and vodka also.

There are also a few supplements you can take, in order to make sure you induce autophagy. You can take nicotinamide and resveratrol. Also known as niacin, nicotinamide is a form of the B3 vitamin. There is also another name to it, NAD+. Nicotinamide is responsible for converting food into energy, repairing the damaged DNA, a stronger cell protection system and also for setting up the circadian rhythm. The RDA for it is around 250-300 mg, and there are plenty of supplements available on the market, to make sure you have the required intake.

Resveratrol is a plant compound which can be used to trigger autophagy. It can be found easily in red grapes, dark chocolate, blueberries, and peanut butter. The recommended daily dosage should be around 250 mg. Your body needs to function properly in order to induce autophagy and in order to make sure it does all its functions as it should, you need to make sure it has the recommended dosage of calcium, magnesium, potassium, omega-3s, iron, vitamin A, the vitamin B group, vitamin C, vitamin D, vitamin E and also vitamin K.

Conclusion

The researches on Autophagy deserved to win the Nobel prize in Physiology or Medicine in 2016, as it's a practice that revolutionizes the medicine. The process of recycling damaged parts or proteins and organelles at a cellular level can have plenty of benefits for the human body, in terms of health, especially. Only when you think of several benefits that autophagy can have, like a better cognitive function (protecting you from neurodegenerative diseases like Alzheimer's and Parkinson's disease), lower blood sugar and insulin level (thus preventing type 2 diabetes), increased ketones level (favoring the fat burning process), appetite control and prevention of heart, kidney, stomach or liver diseases. Around 70% of the diseases known to man are caused by the food we eat, and carbs are playing a major role in favoring diseases. We are too exposed to processed food, and therefore to carbs, so eating healthy it's becoming more of a challenge. In this book, it was already discussed how autophagy could be induced through fasting and the ketosis process. Fasting literally means food abstinence, so you don't have to eat anything in the fasting period. The whole purpose of this process is to burn more fat. As glucose is the default fuel type for the human body, switching the energy source from glucose to fats is something that Intermittent Fasting is aiming for. Glucose is originated from carbs, but since we consume too many carbs and we have a sedentary lifestyle, it doesn't get burned by the body, so it gets stored in the blood, raising the insulin and blood sugar levels. By switching to fats, Intermittent Fasting forces ketones to multiply and to extract the energy from the fat cells. Whilst this happens, the insulin level is getting lower, and it takes care of the blood sugar, regulating it. Ketosis is a phase of Intermittent Fasting during which the ketones levels are significant increases, whilst the blood sugar and insulin level decreases. The Keto-Adaptation process is when the body starts to run on fats as the default fuel type. There are several ways of fasting and even a keto-diet, all of them favoring the autophagy process. However, if fasting is not your thing, you can induce autophagy through HIIT (a really intense workout) or through protein fast, which is a special one-day diet, which involves keeping the daily protein intake to less than 15 grams. Another important piece in the autophagy puzzle is sleep, as autophagy happens during sleep, so without proper restful sleep, the whole process wouldn't take place. Combining all of these factors will get you a lot closer to autophagy.

References

Asprey, Dave. "What Is Bulletproof Protein Fasting & How To Fast Correctly." *Bulletproof*, 12 Dec. 2017, blog.bulletproof.com/what-is-protein-fasting-bulletproof-diet/.

Eenfeldt, Andreas, and Bret Scher. "A Ketogenic Diet for Beginners - The Ultimate Keto Guide." *Diet Doctor*, 7 May 2019, www.dietdoctor.com/low-carb/keto.

Enos, Deborah. "4 Foods That Are Good Sources of Resveratrol." *LiveScience*, Purch, 23 Aug. 2013,

Fung, Jason. "Autophagy – a Cure for Many Present-Day Diseases?" *Diet Doctor*, 19 Dec. 2017, www.dietdoctor.com/autophagy-cure-many-present-day-diseases.

Jarreau, Paige. "The 5 Stages of Intermittent Fasting." *LIFE Apps | LIVE and LEARN*, 10 Apr. 2019, lifeapps.io/fasting/the-5-stages-of-intermittent-fasting/

www.livescience.com/39125-foods-good-sources-resveratrol.html.

Land, S. (2018). *Metabolic autophagy*. Independently Published

Levine, Beth, and Daniel J. Klionsky. "Autophagy Wins the 2016 Nobel Prize in Physiology or Medicine: Breakthroughs in Baker's Yeast Fuel Advances in Biomedical Research." *PNAS*, National Academy of Sciences, 10 Jan. 2017, www.pnas.org/content/114/2/201.

Levy, Jillian. "Benefits of Autophagy, Plus How to Induce It." *Dr. Axe*, 4 Sept. 2018, draxe.com/benefits-of-autophagy/.

Raman, Ryan. "Nicotinamide Riboside: Benefits, Side Effects and Dosage." *Healthline*, Healthline Media, 10 Dec. 2018, www.healthline.com/nutrition/nicotinamide-riboside#what-it-is.

Spritzler, Franziska, and Andreas Eenfeldt. "What Is Ketosis? Is It Safe? – Diet Doctor." *Diet Doctor*, 22 Mar. 2019, www.dietdoctor.com/low-carb/ketosis.

Yang, Zhifen, and Daniel J Klionsky. "Eaten Alive: a History of Macroautophagy." *Nature Cell Biology*, U.S. National Library of Medicine, Sept. 2010, www.ncbi.nlm.nih.gov/pmc/articles/PMC3616322/

---

[i] Yang, Zhifen, and Daniel J Klionsky. "Eaten Alive: a History of Macroautophagy." *Nature Cell Biology*, U.S. National Library of Medicine, Sept. 2010, www.ncbi.nlm.nih.gov/pmc/articles/PMC3616322/.

[ii] Yang, Zhifen, and Daniel J Klionsky. "Eaten Alive: a History of Macroautophagy." *Nature Cell Biology*, U.S. National Library of Medicine, Sept. 2010, www.ncbi.nlm.nih.gov/pmc/articles/PMC3616322/

[iii] Levine, Beth, and Daniel J. Klionsky. "Autophagy Wins the 2016 Nobel Prize in Physiology or Medicine: Breakthroughs in Baker's Yeast Fuel Advances in Biomedical Research." *PNAS*, National Academy of Sciences, 10 Jan. 2017, www.pnas.org/content/114/2/201.

[iv] Levine, Beth, and Daniel J. Klionsky. "Autophagy Wins the 2016 Nobel Prize in Physiology or Medicine: Breakthroughs in Baker's Yeast Fuel Advances in Biomedical Research." *PNAS*, National Academy of Sciences, 10 Jan. 2017, www.pnas.org/content/114/2/201.

[v] Levine, Beth, and Daniel J. Klionsky. "Autophagy Wins the 2016 Nobel Prize in Physiology or Medicine: Breakthroughs in Baker's Yeast Fuel Advances in Biomedical Research." *PNAS*, National Academy of Sciences, 10 Jan. 2017, www.pnas.org/content/114/2/201.

[vi] Levine, Beth, and Daniel J. Klionsky. "Autophagy Wins the 2016 Nobel Prize in Physiology or Medicine: Breakthroughs in Baker's Yeast Fuel Advances in Biomedical Research." *PNAS*, National Academy of Sciences, 10 Jan. 2017, www.pnas.org/content/114/2/201.

[vii] Fung, Jason. "Autophagy – a Cure for Many Present-Day Diseases?" *Diet Doctor*, 19 Dec. 2017, www.dietdoctor.com/autophagy-cure-many-present-day-diseases.

[viii] Land, S. (2018). *Metabolic autophagy.* Independently Published, p.94.

[ix] Land, S. (2018). *Metabolic autophagy.* Independently Published, p.94.

[x] Land, S. (2018). *Metabolic autophagy.*

Independently Published, p.130.

[xi] Land, S. (2018). *Metabolic autophagy.* Independently Published, p. 104

[xii] Land, S. (2018). *Metabolic autophagy.* Independently Published, p. 104

[xiii] Levy, Jillian. "Benefits of Autophagy, Plus How to Induce It." *Dr. Axe*, 4 Sept. 2018, draxe.com/benefits-of-autophagy/.

[xiv] Fung, Jason. "Autophagy – a Cure for Many Present-Day Diseases?" *Diet Doctor*, 19 Dec. 2017, www.dietdoctor.com/autophagy-cure-many-present-day-diseases.

[xv] Land, S. (2018). *Metabolic autophagy.* Independently Published, p. 190

[xvi] Land, S. (2018). *Metabolic autophagy.*

Independently Published, p. 95

[xvii] Spritzler, Franziska, and Andreas Eenfeldt. "What Is Ketosis? Is It Safe? – Diet Doctor." *Diet Doctor*, 22 Mar. 2019, www.dietdoctor.com/low-carb/ketosis.

[xviii] Spritzler, Franziska, and Andreas Eenfeldt. "What Is Ketosis? Is It Safe? – Diet Doctor." *Diet Doctor*, 22 Mar. 2019, www.dietdoctor.com/low-carb/ketosis.

[xix] Eenfeldt, Andreas, and Bret Scher. "A Ketogenic Diet for Beginners - The Ultimate Keto Guide." *Diet Doctor*, 7 May 2019, www.dietdoctor.com/low-carb/keto.

[xx] Land, S. (2018). *Metabolic autophagy.* Independently Published, p. 285

[xxi] Land, S. (2018). *Metabolic autophagy.* Independently Published, p. 286

[xxii] Spritzler, Franziska, and Andreas Eenfeldt. "What Is Ketosis? Is It Safe? – Diet Doctor." *Diet Doctor*, 22 Mar. 2019, www.dietdoctor.com/low-carb/ketosis.

[xxiii] H, Karen, et al. "The 5 Stages of Intermittent Fasting." *LIFE Apps | LIVE and LEARN*, 10 Apr. 2019, lifeapps.io/fasting/the-5-stages-of-intermittent-fasting/.

[xxiv] Jarreau, Paige. "The 5 Stages of Intermittent Fasting." *LIFE Apps | LIVE and LEARN*, 10 Apr. 2019, lifeapps.io/fasting/the-5-stages-of-intermittent-fasting/.

[xxv] Land, S. (2018). *Metabolic autophagy*. Independently Published, p. 126

[xxvi] Asprey, Dave. "What Is Bulletproof Protein Fasting & How To Fast Correctly." *Bulletproof*,

12 Dec. 2017, blog.bulletproof.com/what-is-protein-fasting-bulletproof-diet/.

[xxvii] Asprey, Dave. "What Is Bulletproof Protein Fasting & How To Fast Correctly." *Bulletproof*, 12 Dec. 2017, blog.bulletproof.com/what-is-protein-fasting-bulletproof-diet/.

[xxviii] Asprey, Dave. "What Is Bulletproof Protein Fasting & How To Fast Correctly." *Bulletproof*, 12 Dec. 2017, blog.bulletproof.com/what-is-protein-fasting-bulletproof-diet/.

[xxix] Land, S. (2018). *Metabolic autophagy*. Independently Published, p. 126

[xxx] Land, S. (2018). *Metabolic autophagy*. Independently Published, p. 313

[xxxi] Land, S. (2018). *Metabolic autophagy*. Independently Published, p. 355

[xxxii] Land, S. (2018). *Metabolic autophagy.* Independently Published, p. 355-356

Printed in Poland
by Amazon Fulfillment
Poland Sp. z o.o., Wrocław